Esophageal Disorders

Ronnie Fass · Fahmi Shibli
Michael Kurin · Sherif Saleh
Yoshitaka Kitayama
Editors

Esophageal Disorders

A Clinical Casebook

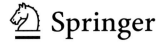

Springer

Editors
Ronnie Fass
Esophageal and Swallowing Center
Case Western Reserve University
Cleveland, OH, USA

Fahmi Shibli
Esophageal and Swallowing Center
Case Western Reserve University
Cleveland, OH, USA

Michael Kurin
Division of Gastroenterology
Case Western Reserve University
Cleveland, OH, USA

Sherif Saleh
Division of Gastroenterology
Case Western Reserve University
Cleveland, OH, USA

Yoshitaka Kitayama
Department of Gastroenterology
Hyogo Medical University Hospital
Nishinomiya, Hyogo, Japan

ISBN 978-3-031-56440-6   ISBN 978-3-031-56441-3   (eBook)
https://doi.org/10.1007/978-3-031-56441-3

This Springer imprint is published by the registered company Springer Nature Switzerland AG
The registered company address is: Gewerbestrasse 11, 6330 Cham, Switzerland

Paper in this product is recyclable.

Preface

Esophageal disorders are very common and are one of the most common reasons for patient visits in the gastroenterology clinic. The last two decades have seen significant developments in esophageal testing and the introduction of several consensus meetings that profoundly shaped the field, especially on how we diagnose and treat esophageal disorders. The latter includes the Chicago Classification, Rome criteria, and Lyon diagnostic metrics for GERD. These important changes in the esophageal field were the impetus behind the development of this case book. In particular, the need to know how to use and interpret the currently available diagnostic techniques and how to incorporate the new proposed consensus guidelines into our clinical practice. Consequently, a group of internal medicine residents under the guidance of Dr. Fahmi Shibli, Dr. Michael Kurin, and I identified interesting and sometimes challenging esophageal cases from the GI function unit at MetroHealth Medical Center. The purpose of this book is to educate the readers about various esophageal disorders through the presentation and discussion of clinically relevant cases. Efforts were made to include original samples of the diagnostic tests that were performed as part of the workup that patients had to undergo. The discussion attempts to critically evaluate the workup and management of the presented patient and offer an overview of the final diagnosis.

This book is intended to serve students, residents, fellows, and faculty from different disciplines with interest in esophageal disorders. I am deeply indebted to the residents who took the time from their busy schedule to summarize these interesting cases and to Michael Kurin, MD, Fahmi Shibli, MD, and Sherif Saleh, MD for helping to edit the content.

This book represents the hard work of many who decided to dedicate a significant part of their free time to improve education in the area of esophageal disorders.

I hope you will enjoy the book and use it to further your understanding of this important area in gastroenterology.

Cleveland, OH, USA   Ronnie Fass, MD, MACG

Contents

Contributors

Subhan Ahmad Division of Hospital Medicine, Case Western Reserve University School of Medicine, MetroHealth Medical Center, Cleveland, OH, USA

Josue Davila Division of Hospital Medicine, Cleveland Clinic Foundation, Cleveland, OH, USA

Sara Ghoneim Department of Gastroenterology and Hepatology, University of Nebraska College of Medicine, University of Nebraska Medical Center, Omaha, NE, USA

Sara Kamionkowski Department of Gastroenterology and Hepatology, Case Western Reserve University School of Medicine, MetroHealth Medical Center, Cleveland, OH, USA

Yeseong Kim Division of Gastroenterology and Hepatology, Lewis Katz School of Medicine at Temple University, Temple University Hospital, Philadelphia, PA, USA

Erika Mengalle Lifespan Physician Group, Division of Hospital Medicine, Warren Alpert Medical School of Brown University, Rhode Island Hospital, Providence, RI, USA

Sherif Saleh Department of Gastroenterology and Hepatology, Case Western Reserve University School of Medicine, MetroHealth Medical Center, Cleveland, OH, USA

Fahmi Shibli Gastroenterology and Liver Diseases, Emek Medical Center, Afula, Israel

Heartburn Without Acid

Yeseong Kim

1   Case Presentation

An 80-year-old male with coronary artery disease, hypertension, and documented gastroesophageal reflux disease (GERD) in the past (Los Angeles grade B erosive esophagitis) presented to clinic for persistent heartburn during both daytime and nighttime despite anti-reflux treatment. The patient also reported that nighttime symptoms are causing him to awaken from sleep during the night. He was also complaining of epigastric pain, nausea, and vomiting. He reported no dysphagia or odynophagia but was having choking episodes after swallows and a change in his voice. An upper endoscopy was unremarkable with no evidence of persistent erosive esophagitis. A modified barium swallow showed mild laryngeal penetration with nectar thickened barium. His anti-reflux regimen at the time consisted of pantoprazole 40 mg daily and ranitidine 300 mg at bedtime. His PPI was increased to twice-daily dosing, and he was referred to ENT for evaluation of oropharyngeal dysphagia. Laryngoscopic evaluation revealed postcricoid edema, thought to be related to GERD, and no other abnormalities. He was referred back to the esophageal clinic, at which point he underwent pH-impedance testing done while on PPI twice a day, which showed normal acidic or weakly acidic reflux, normal reflux burden, and negative symptom association (Table 1). He was diagnosed with functional heartburn. His acid suppression was decreased to PPI once daily, and he was managed with low-dose amitriptyline. He was also referred to psychology for mindfulness coaching. On follow-up, the patient reported complete resolution of symptoms.

Y. Kim (✉)
Division of Gastroenterology and Hepatology, Lewis Katz School of Medicine at Temple University, Temple University Hospital, Philadelphia, PA, USA

© The Author(s), under exclusive license to Springer Nature   1
Switzerland AG 2024
R. Fass et al. (eds.), *Esophageal Disorders*,
https://doi.org/10.1007/978-3-031-56441-3_1

Table 1 Results of the pH-impedance test showing normal amount of acidic and weakly acidic reflux events as well as normal reflux burden an SI

	pH (% time pH <4)
Upright	0.4
Supine	0
Total	0.3

Total number of reflux events

	Acid	Weakly acid	Nonacid	Liquid	Mixed	Total
Upright	2	7	0	4	5	9
Supine	0	0	0	0	0	0
Total	2	7	0	4	5	9

Indices: SI = 0, SAP = 0, *SI* symptom index, *SAP* symptom association probability

2 Discussion

GERD patients with reflux symptoms that do not adequately respond to twice-daily PPI should be further investigated [1]. This patient with previously known GERD presented with refractory GERD symptoms. It is important to note that refractory GERD symptoms can be due to inadequately controlled GERD or due to an overlap with a functional esophageal disorder. Because this patient already had proven GERD, the goal of further testing should focus on determining whether there is evidence of pathologic reflux that persists despite patient's consumption of antisecretory medication. For this reason, reflux testing in this patient population is performed while on high-dose PPI therapy. Since the diagnosis of underlying GERD has already been established, catheter-based pH-impedance testing is preferred over wireless pH capsule testing. The increased sensitivity for detecting GERD offered by the latter is less important in patients with established GERD, and pH-impedance testing provides information pertaining to weakly acid reflux that is helpful for the differentiation between functional esophageal disorders. Functional heartburn (FH) is distinguished from reflux hypersensitivity (RH) by the lack of symptom correlation with any type of reflux events [2, 3].

After a negative upper endoscopy, this patient underwent pH-impedance testing while on PPI twice daily. This test revealed adequately controlled GERD and documented symptoms that did not correlate with reflux events, consistent with GERD that is overlapping with FH. FH is defined as retrosternal burning discomfort or pain refractory to optimal antisecretory therapy in the absence of uncontrolled GERD, histopathologic mucosal abnormalities, major motor disorders, or structural abnormalities [3–5]. When FH presents with underlying GERD, its treatment should include continuation of PPI therapy with the addition of a treatment for FH, which can include neuromodulators and behavioral therapies such as hypnotherapy [4–6].

References

1. Zerbib F, Bredenoord A, Fass R, Kahrilas P, Roman S, Savarino E, Sifrim D, Vaezi M, Yadlapati R, Gyawali C. ESNM/ANMS consensus paper: diagnosis and management of refractory gastro-esophageal reflux disease. Neurogastroenterol Motil. 2020;33(4):e14075.
2. Aziz Q, Fass R, Gyawali CP, Miwa H, Pandolfino JE, Zerbib F. Esophageal disorders. Gastroenterology. 2016;150(6):1368–79.
3. Kondo T, Miwa H. The role of esophageal hypersensitivity in functional heartburn. J Clin Gastroenterol. 2017;51(7):571–8.
4. Fass R. Functional heartburn: what it is and how to treat it. Gastrointest Endosc Clin N Am. 2009;19(1):23–33.
5. Fass R, Tougas G. Functional heartburn: the stimulus, the pain, and the brain. Gut. 2002;51(6):885–92.
6. Riehl ME, Pandolfino JE, Palsson OS, Keefer L. Feasibility and acceptability of esophageal-directed hypnotherapy for functional heartburn. Dis Esophagus. 2016;29(5):490–6.

An Allergic Esophagus?

Yeseong Kim

1   Case Presentation

A 58-year-old professional singer with chronic reflux symptoms, bipolar I disorder, obstructive sleep apnea, allergic rhinitis, and prior deep vein thrombosis presented to the gastroenterology clinic for the evaluation of his chronic reflux symptoms and dysphagia.

The patient reported symptoms of chronic heartburn for which he used to take omeprazole but switched to Tums after symptoms improved. For the past several months, he had been having progressively worsening dysphagia to solid foods with a few episodes of prolonged sensation of bread getting stuck in his chest that eventually subsided after drinking water. These episodes were intermittent and infrequent, occurring once every 1–2 months. There was no dysphagia to liquids. He denied weight loss, vomiting, nausea, abdominal pain, or changes to his appetite. He is a nonsmoker and had no family history of esophageal cancer.

Esophagogastroduodenoscopy (EGD) was performed which showed a small hiatal hernia and multiple fixed concentric esophageal rings that made the inner esophagus appear similar to the trachea (Fig. 1). There were no strictures, masses, exudates, linear furrows, or plaques. Biopsies were taken from the mid-esophagus and showed 20–25 intraepithelial eosinophils per high-power field, consistent with eosinophilic esophagitis (EoE). He was started on omeprazole 40 mg twice a day and was referred to allergy where he underwent skin testing. Based on the results of skin testing, he began excluding egg, corn, soy, wheat, and peanut from his diet. Subsequently, his dysphagia improved. Eight weeks later, the patient returned for repeat endoscopy which showed resolution of the endoscopic findings of concentric

Y. Kim (✉)
Division of Gastroenterology and Hepatology, Lewis Katz School of Medicine at Temple University, Temple University Hospital, Philadelphia, PA, USA

© The Author(s), under exclusive license to Springer Nature Switzerland AG 2024
R. Fass et al. (eds.), *Esophageal Disorders*,
https://doi.org/10.1007/978-3-031-56441-3_2

Fig. 1 Endoscopic image showing esophageal rings in the distal esophagus and proximal esophagus

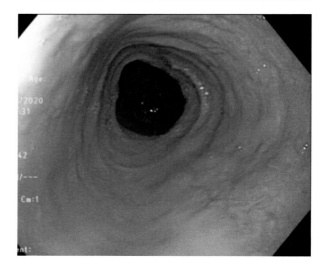

esophageal rings. Biopsies taken from the proximal and distal esophagus showed no eosinophils per high-power field.

2   Discussion

EoE is a chronic immune-mediated inflammatory disease of the esophagus that is defined by symptoms of esophageal dysfunction such as dysphagia or feeding difficulties with an esophageal biopsy demonstrating at least 15 eosinophils per high-power field in the absence of other conditions associated with esophageal eosinophilia [1]. Epidemiological studies show that the incidence of EoE is increasing, with an incidence rate of 43 patients per 100,000 [2]. It most commonly affects young, Caucasian males. Many patients have comorbid atopic disease. Up to 15% of patients evaluated with upper endoscopy for dysphagia are ultimately diagnosed with EoE [3].

The pathophysiology of EoE involves a dysregulated helper T-cell response to environmental antigens causing inappropriate eosinophil recruitment to the esophagus [4]. The most important consideration in the differential diagnosis for EoE is GERD, as acid reflux can cause esophageal eosinophilia as well. Other causes of secondary eosinophilia must be ruled out prior to confirming the diagnosis.

Management of EoE can involve dietary and/or pharmacologic therapy. There are currently three treatment options that are considered first-line therapy: elimination diet, PPIs, and topical steroids [1]. The traditional elimination diet is a six-food elimination diet which includes dairy, wheat, soy, eggs, nuts, and seafood/shellfish [5]. More recent studies have suggested four-food or even two-food elimination diet may have similar efficacy [6]. PPIs may be given with standard dosing of once daily, or twice daily, depending on patient's response. Topical budesonide or fluticasone are the most commonly used topical glucocorticoids. The choice of initial therapy primarily depends on patient preference and several first-line therapies may be combined in the setting of inadequate response to monotherapy [7]. Our patient was referred for allergy testing to guide his elimination diet, a method used by some practitioners that requires more data to determine its efficacy compared to the standard elimination diets.

References

1. Muir A, Falk GW. Eosinophilic esophagitis: a review. JAMA. 2021;326(13):1310–8. https://doi.org/10.1001/jama.2021.14920.
2. Hruz P, Straumann A, Bussmann C, Heer P, Simon H-U, Zwahlen M, et al. Escalating incidence of eosinophilic esophagitis: a 20-year prospective, population-based study in Olten County, Switzerland. J Allergy Clin Immunol. 2011;128(6):1349.
3. Pasha S, DiBaise J, Kim H, De Petris G, Crowell M, Fleischer D, et al. Patient characteristics, clinical, endoscopic, and histologic findings in adult eosinophilic esophagitis: a case series and systematic review of the medical literature. Dis Esophagus. 2007;20(4):311–9.
4. Hogan SP, Mishra A, Brandt EB, Foster PS, Rothenberg ME. A critical role for eotaxin in experimental oral antigen-induced eosinophilic gastrointestinal allergy. Proc Natl Acad Sci. 2000;97(12):6681–6.
5. Molina-Infante J, Arias Á, Alcedo J, Garcia-Romero R, Casabona-Frances S, Prieto-Garcia A, et al. Step-up empiric elimination diet for pediatric and adult eosinophilic esophagitis: the 2-4-6 study. J Allergy Clin Immunol. 2018;141(4):1365–72.
6. Kagalwalla AF, Wechsler JB, Amsden K, et al. Efficacy of a 4-food elimination diet for children with eosinophilic esophagitis. Clin Gastroenterol Hepatol. 2017;15(11):1698–1707.e7.
7. Alexander JA, Jung KW, Arora AS, Enders F, Katzka DA, Kephardt GM, et al. Swallowed fluticasone improves histologic but not symptomatic response of adults with eosinophilic esophagitis. Clin Gastroenterol Hepatol. 2012;10(7):742–9.e1.

Years of Dysphagia

Yeseong Kim

1 Case Presentation

A 79-year-old woman with diverticulosis, atrial fibrillation, hyperlipidemia, hypertension, and obesity presented to gastroenterology clinic for ongoing epigastric pain, heartburn, nausea, and intermittent dysphagia to solids only, which had been ongoing for several years. She reports sensation of having food stuck in the esophagus but denies any vomiting episodes. She also denies any dysphagia to liquids, weight loss, or other oropharyngeal symptoms. She underwent esophagogastroduodenoscopy (EGD) which showed several small gastric ulcers (biopsy was negative for *H. pylori*), small hiatal hernia, and a normal-appearing esophagus. She was placed on a PPI. However, she returned to the clinic with persistent symptoms of dysphagia unresponsive to increasing doses of PPI therapy and was referred for a high-resolution esophageal manometry (HREM). The HREM showed an elevated integrated relaxation pressure (IRP) in both supine and upright swallows with otherwise normal peristalsis and increased intrabolus pressurization consistent with esophagogastric junction outflow obstruction (EGJOO) (Fig. 1, Table 1). Unfortunately, the patient was lost to follow-up after her manometry.

2 Discussion

EGJOO is one of the disorders of the esophageal outlet in which there is obstruction of passage of swallowed contents into the stomach in the absence of a disorder of peristalsis or mechanical obstruction [1–4]. According to the Chicago Classification v4.0, the diagnosis of EGJOO has stringent criteria, in which the elevated IRP must be persistent

Y. Kim (✉)
Division of Gastroenterology and Hepatology, Lewis Katz School of Medicine at Temple University, Temple University Hospital, Philadelphia, PA, USA

R. Fass et al. (eds.), *Esophageal Disorders*,
https://doi.org/10.1007/978-3-031-56441-3_3

9

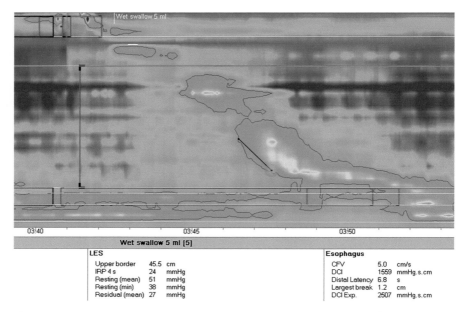

Fig. 1 A representative swallow from high-resolution esophageal manometry showing an elevated integrated relaxation pressure (IRP) with normal peristalsis and increased intrabolus pressurization. Tabular numbers pertain to this particular swallow

Table 1 Aggregate measures of high-resolution esophageal manometry based on ten supine swallows

Indication: Dysphagia	
LES	
Median IRP (mmHg)	20.66
Mean resting pressure (mmHg)	60
Residual pressure (mmHg)	17
UES resting	35
Esophagus	
CFV (cm/s)	3.5
DCI (mmHg s cm)	2863
Distal latency (s)	7.9

during both supine and upright positions and secondary evidence of distal esophageal obstruction such as the finding of increase intrabolus pressurization must be present [1]. Mechanical obstruction must also be excluded, and when no lesion is found on EGD, other forms of imaging such as CT chest and/or endoscopic ultrasound may be recommended. Supportive evidence for EGJOO may be provided by a timed barium esophagram to confirm a functional obstruction and a true delay in emptying of esophageal contents into the stomach as well as the EndoFLIP procedure [1–4].

EGJOO can sometimes be transient, and conservative management with observation and medical therapy for a period of 6 months is recommended in patients with recent onset or mild to moderate symptoms [1, 3]. In addition, opioid consumption should be ruled out as this class of drugs has been shown to be associated with increased IRP [5]. In patients with severe symptoms of dysphagia, treatment of EGJOO is similar to that of achalasia, as both conditions are mediated by failure of LES relaxation. Treatment strategies are aimed to lower LES pressure with endoscopic botulinum toxin injection, surgical myotomy, peroral endoscopic myotomy (POEM), or pneumatic dilation, though data for any of these treatments is not as robust as it is for achalasia [1, 6].

References

1. Yadlapati R, Kahrilas PJ, Fox MR, et al. Esophageal motility disorders on high-resolution manometry: Chicago classification version 4.0©. Neurogastroenterol Motil. 2021;33(1):e14058.
2. Jung KW. [Chicago classification ver. 4.0: diagnosis of achalasia and esophagogastric junction outflow obstruction]. Korean J Gastroenterol. 2022;79(2):61–5. Korean. https://doi.org/10.4166/kjg.2022.017.
3. Samo S, Qayed E. Esophagogastric junction outflow obstruction: where are we now in diagnosis and management? World J Gastroenterol. 2019;25(4):411.
4. Clayton SB, Patel R, Richter JE. Functional and anatomic esophagogastric junction outflow obstruction: manometry, timed barium esophagram findings, and treatment outcomes. Clin Gastroenterol Hepatol. 2016;14(6):907–11.
5. Babaei A, Szabo A, Shad S, Massey BT. Chronic daily opioid exposure is associated with dysphagia, esophageal outflow obstruction, and disordered peristalsis. Neurogastroenterol Motil. 2019;31(7):e13601.
6. Kahrilas PJ, Bredenoord AJ, Fox M, et al. Expert consensus document: advances in the management of oesophageal motility disorders in the era of high-resolution manometry: a focus on achalasia syndromes. Nat Rev Gastroenterol Hepatol. 2017;14:677–88.

When the Band Is Too Tight

Sara Ghoneim

1   Case Presentation

A 50-year-old male was seen in the gastroenterology clinic for the chief complaint of chronic cough. He had suffered several episodes of aspiration pneumonia over the past 1 year. His past medical history is significant for morbid obesity, atrial fibrillation, and type 2 diabetes mellitus. He underwent sleeve gastrectomy 15 years prior which was converted to Roux-en-Y gastric bypass with gastric band placement 18 months later due to inadequate weight loss. Around this time, the patient complained of heartburn and was started on high-dose PPI. He ultimately developed chronic cough and several episodes of aspiration pneumonia prompting extensive pulmonary and cardiac workup that was unrevealing. A barium swallow showed a large volume of gastroesophageal reflux that reaches the level of the thoracic inlet the patient also had evidence of slight irregularity in the distal esophagus (Fig. 1). An upper endoscopy showed a normal-appearing esophagus and gastric remnant without anastomotic ulcers (Fig. 2). He subsequently underwent 24-h ambulatory pH impedance study off PPI which showed a borderline esophageal acid exposure time and an elevated total number of reflux events with positive symptom association (Fig. 3). High-resolution esophageal manometry was performed and revealed a high-pressure zone immediately below the LES, consistent with the location of the gastric band (Fig. 4). It was felt the patient had an esophagogastric junction outlet obstruction due to the band. The patient underwent laparoscopic removal of the gastric band with resolution of his cough.

S. Ghoneim (✉)
Department of Gastroenterology and Hepatology, University of Nebraska College of
Medicine, University of Nebraska Medical Center, Omaha, NE, USA

© The Author(s), under exclusive license to Springer Nature
Switzerland AG 2024
R. Fass et al. (eds.), *Esophageal Disorders*,
https://doi.org/10.1007/978-3-031-56441-3_4

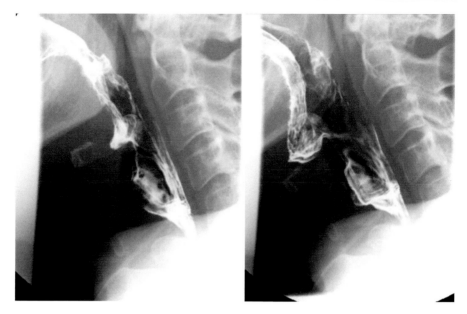

Fig. 1 Barium swallow showing large volume of gastroesophageal reflux to the level of the thoracic inlet with evidence of slight irregularity in the distal esophagus

Fig. 2 Upper endoscopy with normal-appearing distal esophagus and gastric remnant without mucosal abnormalities

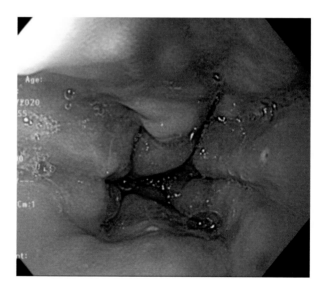

Fig. 3 pH impedance test showing a borderline amount of esophageal acid exposure and an elevated number of reflux events with positive symptom association

1.) pH

Fraction Time pH < 4 (%)

Upright	Supine	Total
4.3	5.3	4.8

2.) Impedance

Total number of reflux events

	Acid	Weakly acid	Non acid	Liquid	Mixed	Total
Upright	39	35	0	26	48	74
Supine	9	6	0	9	6	15
Total	48	41	0	35	54	89

Indices :

SI   44.4%

SAP   99.8%

Esophageal acid Exposure – inconclusive
Weakly Acidic Reflux – borderline
Symptom Indexes – abnormal SAP
Reflux burden – abnormal

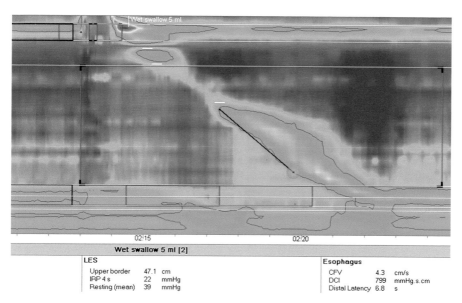

LES			Esophagus		
Upper border	47.1	cm	CFV	4.3	cm/s
IRP 4 s	22	mmHg	DCI	799	mmHg.s.cm
Resting (mean)	39	mmHg	Distal Latency	6.8	s

Fig. 4 A representative swallow from high-resolution esophageal manometry showing a high-pressure zone immediately below the LES. Tabular number below represents the manometric measurements for this representative swallow

2   Discussion

Esophagogastric junction outflow obstruction (EGJOO) is a symptomatic delay in the transit of food through the esophagogastric junction (EGJ) to the stomach. When this occurs in the absence of anatomic obstruction, it represents an esophagogastric function disorder. In our case, the patient had an esophageal outlet obstruction due to mechanical compression after he underwent laparoscopic gastric banding. This case demonstrates the importance of carefully ruling out mechanical obstruction prior to confirming the diagnosis of EGJOO according to the Chicago 4.0 classification [1–3]. Even in the setting of a normal upper endoscopy, further imaging such as chest CT or even endoscopic ultrasound of the EGJ may be considered to ensure no anatomic abnormality is missed. In our case, the surgical history provided the essential clue to the cause of the obstruction.

Among the etiologies of non-functional EGJOO, anatomic causes and hiatal hernia are the most common conditions reported [4, 5]. Management of EGJOO relies on accurate diagnosis and treatment of the underlying etiology. Relief of the mechanical obstruction generally improves the symptoms in patients in whom an anatomic abnormality is identified, as happened in our case.

References

1. Yadlapati R, Kahrilas PJ, Fox MR, et al. Esophageal motility disorders on high-resolution manometry: Chicago classification version 4.0©. Neurogastroenterol Motil. 2021;33(1):e14058. https://doi.org/10.1111/nmo.14058.
2. Jung KW. [Chicago classification ver. 4.0: diagnosis of achalasia and esophagogastric junction outflow obstruction]. Korean J Gastroenterol. 2022;79(2):61–5. Korean.
3. Bredenoord AJ, Babaei A, Carlson D, Omari T, Akiyama J, Yadlapati R, Pandolfino JE, Richter J, Fass R. Esophagogastric junction outflow obstruction. Neurogastroenterol Motil. 2021;33(9):e14193. https://doi.org/10.1111/nmo.14193. Epub 2021 Jun 12.
4. Richter JE, Clayton SB. Diagnosis and management of esophagogastric junction outflow obstruction. Am J Gastroenterol. 2019;114(4):544–7.
5. DeLay K, Austin GL, Menard-Katcher P. Anatomic abnormalities are common potential explanations of manometric esophagogastric junction outflow obstruction. Neurogastroenterol Motil. 2016;28(8):1166–71.

Intractable Nausea and Vomiting in a Patient with Systemic Sclerosis

Sara Kamionkowski

1 Case Presentation

A 67-year-old female with a history of scleroderma complicated by pulmonary hypertension and interstitial lung disease presented to the gastroenterology clinic with complaints of intractable nausea and vomiting of solid foods, after recently suffering a small bowel obstruction. Her vomiting primarily occurred up to 1 h after eating and was associated with epigastric abdominal pain. She had been taking omeprazole without relief. An upper endoscopy was unremarkable (Fig. 1); however, CT enterography showed a distended and fluid-filled distal esophagus, stomach, and small bowel loops (Fig. 2). Gastric emptying study was normal with 3% retained contents at 4 h. High-resolution esophageal manometry (HREM) showed a normal integrated relaxation pressure (IRP), a hypotensive lower esophageal sphincter (LES), and 100% failed swallows (Fig. 3). She was advised to eat small frequent meals and increase her PPI to twice daily. With adherence to these recommendations, she had improvement in her symptoms.

S. Kamionkowski (✉)
Department of Gastroenterology and Hepatology, Case Western Reserve University School of Medicine, MetroHealth Medical Center, Cleveland, OH, USA
e-mail: skamionkowski@metrohealth.org

R. Fass et al. (eds.), *Esophageal Disorders*,
https://doi.org/10.1007/978-3-031-56441-3_5

Fig. 1 Unremarkable
upper endoscopy

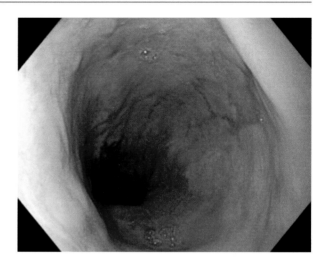

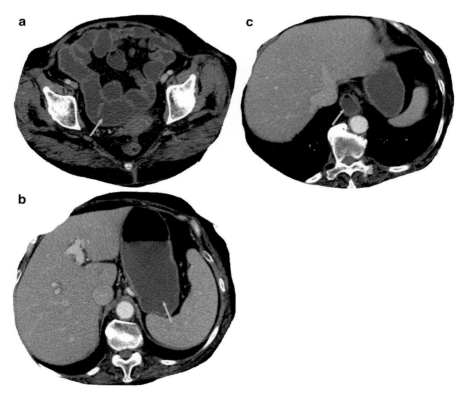

Fig. 2 CT enterography with dilated fluid-filled small bowel loops (**a**), stomach (**b**) and esophagus (**c**)

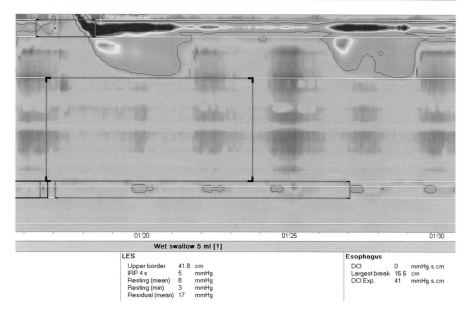

LES				Esophagus		
Upper border	41.8	cm		DCI	0	mmHg.s.cm
IRP 4 s	5	mmHg		Largest break	16.6	cm
Resting (mean)	8	mmHg		DCI Exp.	41	mmHg.s.cm
Resting (min)	3	mmHg				
Residual (mean)	17	mmHg				

Fig. 3 A representative swallow from high-resolution esophageal manometry showing a normal integrated relaxation pressure (IRP), a hypotensive lower esophageal sphincter (LES), and a failed swallow. Tabular numbers below pertain to this representative swallow

2   Discussion

This patient presented with scleroderma esophagus, an absent contractility that is limited to the smooth muscle part of the esophagus. Patients with scleroderma often present with dysphagia or GERD symptoms such as heartburn and regurgitation. However, patients can also present with nausea and vomiting as the primary symptom, as was the case with our patient. This is because the disease involves the smooth muscle of other parts of the GI tract. Patients with scleroderma may also present with normal or ineffective esophageal motility [1, 2]. The pathophysiology of scleroderma is fibrosis of the lamina propria and inhibition of pro-cholinergic enteric neurotransmission. A hypotensive lower esophageal sphincter (LES) is often noted as well. The combination of a weakened gastroesophageal junction barrier with defects in primary and secondary peristalsis makes scleroderma esophagus a very difficult disorder to treat [2, 3].

Workup of patients with esophageal symptoms and a history of scleroderma should include an upper endoscopy, which may reveal complications of GERD or a dilated esophagus with impaired contractions and an open LES [3]. When an esophageal motility disorder is suspected, HREM is the test of choice and will often show absent contractility or ineffective esophageal motility that spares the proximal esophagus [4].

Management of absent contractility, or ineffective esophageal motility in a patient with scleroderma is primarily symptomatic with the goal of improving quality of life and preventing complications of GERD like peptic stricture. This includes aggressive acid suppression with high-dose PPI and lifestyle modifications measures such as elevating the head of bed and avoiding reclining as much as possible. Our patient improved with the aforementioned measures.

References

1. Denton CP, Khanna D. Systemic sclerosis. Lancet. 2017;390(10103):1685–99. https://doi. org/10.1016/S0140-6736(17)30933-9.
2. Frech TM, Mar D. Gastrointestinal and hepatic disease in systemic sclerosis. Rheum Dis Clin N Am. 2018;44(1):15–28. https://doi.org/10.1016/j.rdc.2017.09.002.
3. Fulp SR, Castell DO. Scleroderma esophagus. Dysphagia. 1990;5(4):204–10. https://doi. org/10.1007/BF02412688.
4. Aggarwal N, Lopez R, Gabbard S, Wadhwa N, Devaki P, Thota PN. Spectrum of esophageal dysmotility in systemic sclerosis on high-resolution esophageal manometry as defined by Chicago classification. Dis Esophagus. 2017;30(12):1–6. https://doi.org/10.1093/dote/dox067.

Trouble Swallowing and Blue Fingers

Sherif Saleh

1 Case Presentation

A 57-year-old female with a past medical history of hypothyroidism (status post thyroidectomy), obstructive sleep apnea, and chronic reflux symptoms came to the esophageal clinic after 15 years with progressive dysphagia including two choking episodes requiring Heimlich maneuver with expulsion of partially digested bread. Fifteen years prior she had an esophagogastroduodenoscopy (EGD) with biopsies notable only for LA grade A erosive esophagitis and a nonobstructive Schatzki's ring. A catheter-based pH test demonstrated normal esophageal acid exposure. Her symptoms had been controlled with standard-dose PPI until the past several months.

EGD was performed and showed a 3 cm hiatal hernia with mild gastritis within the hernia sac (Fig. 1) and a nonobstructive Schatzki's ring (Fig. 2). High-resolution esophageal manometry (HREM) was performed, and the results are shown in Fig. 3. The HREM revealed a normal median integrated relaxation pressure (IRP), a hypotensive lower esophageal sphincter (LES) resting pressure, and 100% failed swallows. She was diagnosed with absent contractility. A subsequent barium esophagram showed dilated, aperistaltic esophagus with a patulous gastroesophageal junction (Fig. 4). Upon further questioning she was noted to have Raynaud's phenomenon. After referral to rheumatology, she was ultimately diagnosed with scleroderma. She improved with aggressive acid suppression using twice-daily PPI and a histamine-2 receptor antagonist at bedtime.

S. Saleh (✉)
Department of Gastroenterology and Hepatology, Case Western Reserve University School of Medicine, MetroHealth Medical Center, Cleveland, OH, USA
e-mail: ssaleh1@metrohealth.org

Fig. 1 Endoscopic image of the gastroesophageal junction displaying a small hiatal hernia

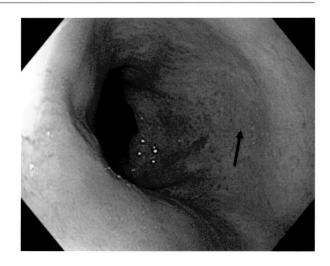

Fig. 2 Endoscopic image of nonobstructive Schatzki's ring

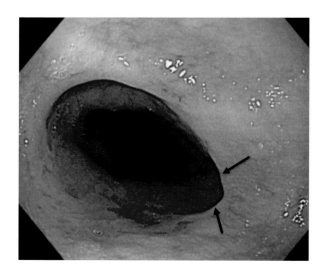

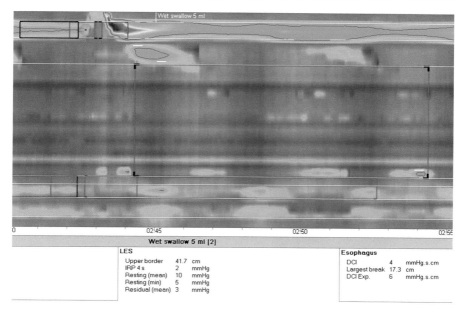

LES			Esophagus		
Upper border	41.7	cm	DCI	4	mmHg.s.cm
IRP 4 s	2	mmHg	Largest break	17.3	cm
Resting (mean)	10	mmHg	DCI Exp.	6	mmHg.s.cm
Resting (min)	5	mmHg			
Residual (mean)	3	mmHg			

Fig. 3 A representative swallow from high-resolution esophageal manometry showing a failed swallow with normal median integrated relaxation pressure and a hypotensive lower esophageal sphincter. Tabular numbers below pertain to this representative swallow

Fig. 4 Barium esophagram showing dilated and aperistaltic esophagus

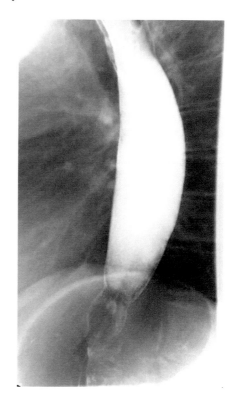

2 Discussion

The esophagus is the most frequently involved portion of the gastrointestinal tract in systemic sclerosis (SSc), with an estimated incidence rate of 40% to 80% [1]. GERD and hypocontractile esophageal motility disorders are the most frequent conditions [2]. Absent contractility, which was previously referred to as "scleroderma esophagus," is a disorder of esophageal peristalsis and is defined by manometry findings of normal IRP with 100% failed swallows. Our patient's clinical history and HREM findings are consistent with the diagnosis of absent contractility. Patients with SSc and absent contractility have absent peristalsis in the distal two-thirds of the esophagus and poor bolus transit that may be seen on esophageal manometry and pH impedance, as well as low or absent LES pressure [3]. In scleroderma, the proximal esophagus (striated muscle) is spared.

As was the case with our patient, esophageal symptoms can be the initial presentation of a systemic disorder such as scleroderma. While a full rheumatologic workup is not immediately recommended for all patients with absent contractility, a careful history and physical exam should be used to look for suggestive signs that would warrant further testing. In our patient, identification of Raynaud's phenomenon triggered the additional workup that eventually led to a diagnosis of systemic sclerosis. It is important to note that absent contractility is not unique to scleroderma and can be seen with other connective tissue disorders, including systemic lupus erythematous, Sjogren syndrome, polymyositis, dermatomyositis, and amyloidosis [4].

There is no specific treatment available for absent contractility [5]. Management is primarily symptomatic with the goal of improving quality of life and includes lifestyle modifications, acid suppression, and when required, antireflux procedures. In this patient, her symptoms improved after starting on a twice-daily PPI and a histamine-2-recepotr antagonist at bedtime.

References

1. Pattanaik D, Brown M, Postlethwaite BC, Postlethwaite AE. Pathogenesis of systemic sclerosis. Front Immunol. 2015;6:272.
2. Denaxas K, Ladas SD, Karamanolis GP. Evaluation and management of esophageal manifestations in systemic sclerosis. Ann Gastroenterol. 2018;31(2):165–70.
3. Yarze JC, Varga J, Stampfl D, Castell DO, Jimenez SA. Esophageal function in systemic sclerosis: a prospective evaluation of motility and acid reflux in 36 patients. Am J Gastroenterol. 1993;88(6):870.
4. Laique S, Singh T, Dornblaser D, Gadre A, Rangan V, Fass R, Kirby D, Chatterjee S, Gabbard S. Clinical characteristics and associated systemic diseases in patients with esophageal "absent contractility"—a clinical algorithm. J Clin Gastroenterol. 2019;53(3):184–90.
5. Ghani S, et al. Esophageal motility disorders in systemic sclerosis. PAMJ Clin Med. 2020;2:108.

Difficulty Swallowing in a Patient with Scleroderma

Sherif Saleh

1 Case Description

A 61-year-old Caucasian woman with scleroderma, anxiety, depression, tobacco use, hypothyroidism, and heartburn presented to the esophageal clinic for evaluation of 6 months of dysphagia to solids and globus sensation. She had a family history of gastric cancer.

She described her dysphagia as heaviness in the throat after eating large solid meals, which resolves after drinking water. She did not have food impaction, regurgitation, or vomiting. She denied dysphagia to liquids, nausea, anorexia, or weight loss. She is taking PPI daily. A barium esophagram was obtained revealing an external compression at the level of the cervical spine (Fig. 1). CT head neck revealed a 3 mm cervical osteophyte without evidence of compression on the esophagus. Esophagogastroduodenoscopy (EGD) showed no esophageal abnormality (Fig. 2). A high-resolution esophageal manometry (HREM) was then performed, demonstrating a normal integrated relaxation pressure (IRP) and 80% weak swallows, suggesting ineffective esophageal motility (IEM) (Fig. 3).

S. Saleh (✉)
Department of Gastroenterology and Hepatology, Case Western Reserve University School of Medicine, MetroHealth Medical Center, Cleveland, OH, USA
e-mail: ssaleh1@metrohealth.org

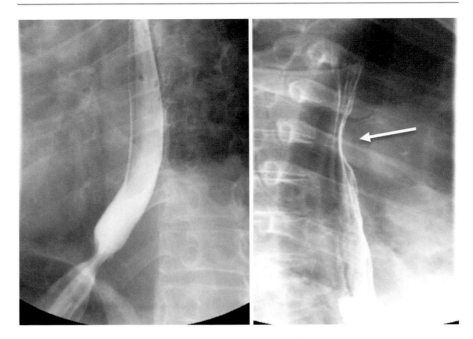

Fig. 1 Barium esophagram showing extrinsic compression

Fig. 2 Upper endoscopy
showing normal
esophageal mucosa

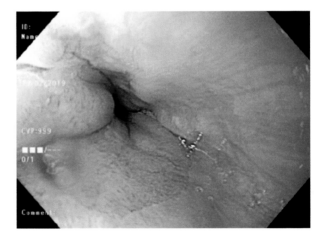

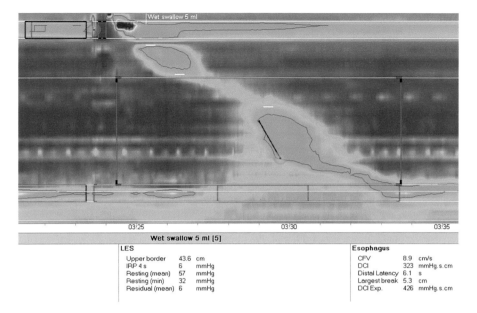

Wet swallow 5 ml [5]				
LES			**Esophagus**	
Upper border	43.6 cm		CFV	8.9 cm/s
IRP 4 s	6 mmHg		DCI	323 mmHg.s.cm
Resting (mean)	57 mmHg		Distal Latency	6.1 s
Resting (min)	32 mmHg		Largest break	5.3 cm
Residual (mean)	6 mmHg		DCI Exp.	426 mmHg.s.cm

Fig. 3 A representative swallow from high-resolution esophageal manometry showing a weak swallow with a normal integrated relaxation pressure. Tabular numbers below pertain to this representative swallow

2 Discussion

The most common gastrointestinal (GI) symptoms in scleroderma patients are GERD-related and dysphagia, as described by this patient. Scleroderma is traditionally associated with absent contractility, but HREM can also reveal IEM as was the case with our patient. According to Chicago 4.0 criteria, IEM is diagnosed when 70% of the swallows are weak (DCI 100–450 mmHg cm s) or 50% are failed (DCI <100 mmHg cm s) [1]. In this case, our patient had an HREM with 80% weak swallows (DCI 323 mmHg cm s) (Fig. 3), which is consistent with IEM. Scleroderma is a chronic immune-mediated multisystem disease with clinical features including cutaneous involvement (sclerodactyly), pulmonary hypertension, interstitial lung disease, Raynaud's phenomenon, and esophageal involvement [2]. The GI tract is involved in up to 90% of the patients with scleroderma. The pathogenesis of IEM in scleroderma likely involves smooth muscle atrophy of the esophageal wall due to collagen deposition and subintimal arterial fibrosis [3, 4].

Upper endoscopy findings in patients with scleroderma include reflux esophagitis, infectious esophagitis, Barrett's esophagus, and esophageal stricture. Erosive esophagitis has been reported in up to 60% of patients with scleroderma and Barrett's metaplasia in more than one-third of these patients [5]. Our patient's upper endoscopy showed no esophageal abnormality. Thus, she was referred for an HREM.

Currently, there is no specific management for IEM or scleroderma. However, treatment focuses on GERD, including acid suppression using a PPI and lifestyle modifications such as elevating the head of bed [6].

References

1. Yadlapati R, Kahrilas PJ, Fox MR, et al. Esophageal motility disorders on high-resolution manometry: Chicago classification version 4.0©. Neurogastroenterol Motil. 2021;33(1):e14058.
2. Denton CP, Khanna D. Systemic sclerosis. Lancet. 2017;390(10103):1685–99. https://doi.org/10.1016/S0140-6736(17)30933-9.
3. Sjogren RW. Gastrointestinal motility disorders in scleroderma. Arthritis Rheum. 1994;37(9):1265–82.
4. Yekeler E, Gürsan N. Esophagectomy in scleroderma: report of a case. Case Rep Gastroenterol. 2008;2(3):499–504.
5. Katzka DA, Reynolds JC, Saul SH, et al. Barrett's metaplasia and adenocarcinoma of the esophagus in scleroderma. Am J Med. 1987;82:46.
6. Ghani S, et al. Esophageal motility disorders in systemic sclerosis. PAMJ Clin Med. 2020;2:108.

Recurrent Episodes of Regurgitation

Sara Kamionkowski

1 Case Presentation

A 28-year-old female with a history of postural orthostatic tachycardia syndrome (POTS) and Ehlers-Danlos syndrome presented to gastroenterology clinic for continued management of long-standing dysphagia, nausea, and vomiting. She initially started having problems with recurrent nausea and vomiting at the age of 15. Her main complaints included sensation of dry foods sticking in throat and choking and regurgitation after initiating a swallow. EGD at the time showed mild gastritis. She also had a normal gastric emptying study and a barium swallow that showed a tablet lodged in the mid-esophagus. A pH impedance test was also normal. She was evaluated by ENT, and laryngoscopy was normal. Her symptoms persisted despite treatment with high-dose pantoprazole prompting further testing with high-resolution esophageal manometry (HREM). Her findings did not meet criteria for an esophageal motility disorder, but she demonstrated several episodes of post-swallow decrease in intraesophageal pressure, consistent with rumination events (Fig. 1). She was diagnosed with rumination syndrome. The patient was referred to speech therapy for diaphragmatic breathing exercises and continued taking pantoprazole.

2 Discussion

Our patient is an example of a common mischaracterization of symptoms, in which rumination evens are inaccurately described as dysphagia or vomiting. Rumination events are often mistaken for reflux events as well. Rumination syndrome is a

S. Kamionkowski (✉)
Department of Gastroenterology and Hepatology, Case Western Reserve University School of Medicine, MetroHealth Medical Center, Cleveland, OH, USA
e-mail: skamionkowski@metrohealth.org

© The Author(s), under exclusive license to Springer Nature Switzerland AG 2024
R. Fass et al. (eds.), *Esophageal Disorders*,
https://doi.org/10.1007/978-3-031-56441-3_8

29

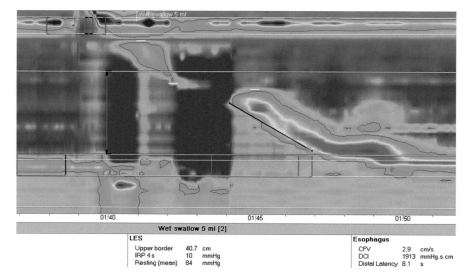

LES			Esophagus		
Upper border	40.7	cm	CFV	2.9	cm/s
IRP 4 s	10	mmHg	DCI	1913	mmHg.s.cm
Resting (mean)	84	mmHg	Distal Latency	8.1	s

Fig. 1 A representative swallow from high-resolution esophageal manometry demonstrating post-swallow decrease in intraesophageal pressure with concomitant increase in intragastric pressure suggestive of rumination event. Tabular numbers pertain to this particular swallow

disorder of gut-brain interaction that is thought to affect 0.8% of the population. It is most prevalent in patients with eating disorders and fibromyalgia [1]. Rumination events are characterized by retrograde flow of undigested gastric contents into the esophagus due to a transient increase in intragastric pressure and decrease in intra-esophageal pressure. Therefore, patients typically present with bland regurgitation that occurs postprandially without preceding nausea. Other symptoms that patients may also experience include heartburn, belching, and bloating. Rumination is often mistaken for GERD due to some similarity of symptoms.

Rumination can be diagnosed clinically, based on the typical description of episodes mentioned above. However, objective testing can be used to support the diagnosis. The test of choice is often HREM. Gastric pressures are often noted to rise above 30 mmHg, which is higher than the intrathoracic esophageal pressure [2]. Esophageal impedance testing can also demonstrate episodes of regurgitation of gastric contents.

Treatment usually involves behavioral modifications. Diaphragmatic breathing techniques with or without biofeedback have been reported to be successful in multiple case reports by augmenting abdominal wall relaxation [3]. Others behavioral techniques that have been used for the treatment of rumination include distraction, cognitive behavioral therapy, and aversion therapy [4]. More randomized controlled trials are needed to compare the different behavioral techniques including diaphragmatic breathing as there is insufficient evidence to show superiority of one method over another. There is no high-quality evidence to support any particular pharmacologic therapy for rumination syndrome, but PPIs, prokinetics, antiemetics, Tricyclic antidepressants, and H2 blockers are often used with unclear efficacy. One study compared baclofen 10 mg three times daily to placebo and demonstrated that baclofen led to greater improvement in symptoms subjects with lower frequency of regurgitation [5].

References

1. Halland M, Pandolfino J, Barba E. Diagnosis and treatment of rumination syndrome. Clin Gastroenterol Hepatol. 2018;16(10):1549–55. https://doi.org/10.1016/j.cgh.2018.05.049.
2. Absah I, Rishi A, Talley NJ, Katzka D, Halland M. Rumination syndrome: pathophysiology, diagnosis, and treatment. Neurogastroenterol Motil. 2017;29(4) https://doi.org/10.1111/nmo.12954.
3. Tack J, Blondeau K, Boecxstaens V, et al. Review article: The pathophysiology, differential diagnosis and management of rumination syndrome. Aliment Pharmacol Ther. 2011;33:782–8.
4. Murray HB, Juarascio AS, Di Lorenzo C, Drossman DA, Thomas JJ. Diagnosis and treatment of rumination syndrome: a critical review. Am J Gastroenterol. 2019;114(4):562–78. https://doi.org/10.14309/ajg.0000000000000060.
5. Pauwels A, Broers C, Van Houtte B, Rommel N, Vanuytsel T, Tack J. A randomized double-blind, placebo-controlled, cross-over study using baclofen in the treatment of rumination syndrome. Am J Gastroenterol. 2018;113(1):97–104. https://doi.org/10.1038/ajg.2017.441.

Fainting While Eating

Fahmi Shibli

1 Case Presentation

An 86-year-old male with coronary artery disease, prior coronary artery bypass graft (CABG), congestive heart failure, atrial fibrillation, hypertension, and a history of gastric ulcer presented to the esophageal clinic for episodes of fainting that occurred during eating. The patient reported developing dysphagia to solids and pills, but not to liquids, soon after his CABG. His dysphagia symptoms progressed after suffering several transient ischemic attacks and a pontine ischemic stroke. Subsequently, he began experiencing syncopal episodes during meals, which resulted in avoidance of socializing and the need to use a safety helmet during meals. The syncopal episodes occurred four times over the span of 2 months, and each was associated with choking and coughing spells prior to fainting, without any other prodromal symptoms. He also reported weight loss due to his dysphagia, but no odynophagia, hoarseness, or chronic cough. A modified barium swallow was performed with speech pathology evaluation, revealing normal oral and pharyngeal phases of swallow. He also underwent an upper endoscopy, which showed no esophageal abnormality. He was evaluated by otolaryngology and had laryngoscopy which showed no abnormality. A high-resolution esophageal manometry (HREM) was then performed and showed normal esophageal motility.

Given the unrevealing workup of his esophagus, the patient was referred to cardiology for evaluation for possible cardiac arrhythmia. He had a Holter monitor placed, revealing bradycardia that precipitated the syncopal episodes that patient experienced while swallowing. A cardiac pacemaker was placed. Subsequently, a barium esophagram was performed demonstrating dilation of the proximal third of the esophagus (Fig. 1). A follow-up computed tomography (CT) of the chest revealed a dilation of the esophagus proximal to the carina due to extrinsic

F. Shibli (✉)
Gastroenterology and Liver Diseases, Emek Medical Center, Afula, Israel

R. Fass et al. (eds.), *Esophageal Disorders*,
https://doi.org/10.1007/978-3-031-56441-3_9

Fig. 1 Barium esophagogram demonstrating dilation of the proximal third of the esophagus

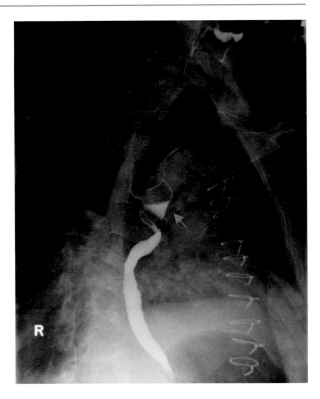

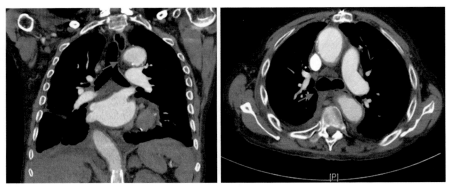

Fig. 2 CT chest with and without contrast showing dilation of the esophagus due to extrinsic compression from a large descending thoracic aortic aneurysm

compression from a large descending thoracic aortic aneurysm (Fig. 2). The patient was diagnosed with deglutitive syncope (DS) due to aortic aneurism (dysphagia aortica) that induced a cardiac arrhythmia. Although the patient was not a candidate for aneurism repair, he did experience a marked reduction in the number of DS episodes after pacemaker placement.

2 Discussion

Deglutitive syncope (DS) is an exceedingly rare condition with less than 100 cases reported in the literature since it was first described over 200 years ago [1]. Approximately 40% of cases have been attributed to underlying digestive disorders, such as hiatal hernia, esophageal stricture, achalasia, and esophageal carcinoma [2, 3]. The majority of syncopal episodes can be explained by abnormal vasovagal stimulation or cardiogenic causes such as sinus bradycardia, arrhythmia, or high degree atrioventricular blocks [2]. The mechanism behind DS involves inappropriate activation of the vagal nerve fibers which connect the esophagus and the heart, resulting in atrioventricular block and a sudden reduction in cardiac output leading to syncope [4]. The stimulus for generating vagal impulses varies widely and includes bolus transit through the esophagus causing mechanical dilation, achalasia, esophageal stricture, esophageal carcinoma, presence of hiatal hernia, and even cold water [5–7].

Initial workup of DS involves a comprehensive evaluation to rule out conventional causes of syncope. This may be achieved by obtaining an electrocardiogram, echocardiogram, tilt-table test, Holter monitor, carotid artery Doppler ultrasound, brain magnetic resonance imaging (MRI), exercise stress test, or a cardiac catheterization. Thorough evaluation for an esophageal disorder is also appropriate, including barium esophagram, upper endoscopy, reflux testing, and HREM. As in our case, imaging studies including CT of the chest are reasonable when considering extraluminal causes of DS.

Treatment of DS is directed toward management of the underlying cause, including avoidance of trigger foods and proper management of esophageal or cardiac disease. Medications such as beta-blockers or calcium channel blockers should be discontinued if possible to downregulate vagal activation and increase cardiac output [8].

This case is unique because we present dysphagia aortica (DA) as a cause of DS. DA in itself is an uncommon cause of dysphagia. DA develops due to a large, atherosclerotic, tortuous, or aneurysmal aorta which causes extrinsic compression or impingement on the esophagus [9]. Management is surgical in patients who are surgical candidates. Patients who are not surgical candidates can attempt non-pharmacologic measures such as eating soft or liquid diet, chewing food carefully, and waiting between swallows. When this is not successful, PEG tube placement may be required.

References

1. Major RH. Classic descriptions of disease: with biographical sketches of the authors. Charles C Thomas Pub Limited; 1945.
2. Mitra S, Ludka T, Rezkalla SH, Sharma PP, Luo J. Swallow syncope: a case report and review of the literature. Clin Med Res. 2011;9(3–4):125–9.
3. Omi W, Murata Y, Yaegashi T, Inomata J-I, Fujioka M, Muramoto S. Swallow syncope, a case report and review of the literature. Cardiology. 2006;105(2):75–9.
4. Siew KSW, Tan MP, Hilmi IN, et al. Swallow syncope: a case report and review of literature. BMC Cardiovasc Disord. 2019;19:191.
5. Bortolotti M, Cirignotta F, Labò G. Atrioventricular block induced by swallowing in a patient with diffuse esophageal spasm. JAMA. 1982;248(18):2297–9.
6. Tomlinson I, Fox K. Carcinoma of the oesophagus with "swallow syncope". Br Med J. 1975;2(5966):315.
7. Trujillo N. Syncope associated with esophageal stricture. Med Ann Dist Columbia. 1974;43(11):553–6.
8. Kang KH, Cho WH, Kim MC, Chang HJ, Chung JI, Won DJ. Cases of swallow syncope induced by the activation of mechanorecepters in the lower esophagus. Korean J Intern Med. 2005;20(1):68.
9. Wilkinson J, Euinton H, Smith L, Bull M, Thorpe J. Diagnostic dilemmas in dysphagia aortica. Eur J Cardiothorac Surg. 1997;11(2):222–7.

The Patient Who Could Not Stop Belching

Fahmi Shibli

1 Case Presentation

A 65-year-old female with no significant past medical history was seen in our gastroenterology clinic for frequent belching that was ongoing for several years. She would constantly try to suppress her belching when in public, but in private she would belch every few minutes. Additionally, she described a pressure-like sensation and burning in her throat. She explained that the more she belched, the worse the burning got. The belching was not associated with eating or any specific foods, and in fact eating made her symptoms improve for about 20 minutes. She did not experience heartburn, regurgitation, nausea, vomiting, abdominal pain, fever, or chills.

An upper endoscopy was performed and was unremarkable. Reflux testing was done with a 48-h wireless pH monitoring. The test was unremarkable with esophageal acid exposure time <4% on day 1 and day 2. High-resolution esophageal manometry (HREM) was performed and showed normal median IRP, normal lower esophageal sphincter (LES) resting pressure, and 100% normal swallows (Fig. 1). Ultimately, she underwent a pH impedance study that again showed normal esophageal acid exposure in both supine and upright positions, no increased number of reflux events (Fig. 2) but with evidence for multiple supragastric belching events. She was diagnosed with supragastric belching and referred for diaphragmatic breathing treatment with improvement in her symptoms.

F. Shibli (✉)
Gastroenterology and Liver Diseases, Emek Medical Center, Afula, Israel

R. Fass et al. (eds.), *Esophageal Disorders*,
https://doi.org/10.1007/978-3-031-56441-3_10

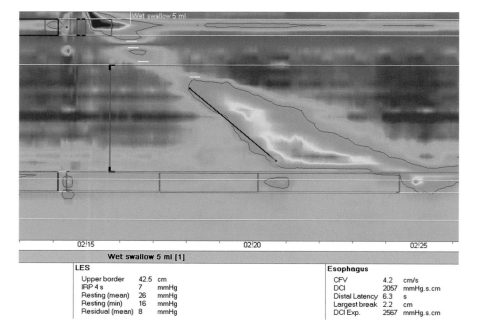

Fig. 1 A representative swallow from high-resolution esophageal manometry demonstrating a normal swallow with normal integrated relaxation pressure. Tabular numbers below pertain to this swallow

1. PH (% time pH <4)

Upright	2.3
Supine	0.5
Total	1.4

2. Impedance

Total number of reflux events

	Acid	Weakly acid	Non acid	Liquid	Mixed	Total
Upright	23	15	0	6	32	38
Supine	2	1	0	2	1	3
Total	25	16	0	8	33	41

3) Indices

SI   0

SAP   0

Fig. 2 pH impedance demonstrating a normal esophageal acid exposure in both supine and upright positions with no increased number of reflux events

2   Discussion

Belching, or eructation, is the escape of air from the esophagus or the stomach into the pharynx. Belching is only considered a disorder when it is excessive and becomes troublesome. Depending on the origin of the refluxed gas, belching is classified into two types: supragastric (esophageal) and gastric belching.

In supragastric belching, patients relax their upper esophageal sphincter, swallow air, and then release it from the esophagus before it reaches the stomach [1]. Swallowing of air into the esophagus may occur by creating a negative intrathoracic pressure and then relaxing the upper esophageal sphincter [2].

According to the Rome IV criteria, pathologic belching is defined as bothersome belching more than 3 days a week [3]. The diagnosis of supragastric belching is supported by observing frequent, repetitive belching that originate from the esophagus. As in our case, esophageal impedance testing can be used to distinguish supragastric from gastric belching, by visualizing the spike in impedance pressure as it travels down and then back up the esophagus without entering the stomach.

Management of supragastric belching includes education to decrease air swallowing and reassurance that belching is a benign condition. Specific behavioral measures include avoidance of gum chewing, smoking, drinking carbonated beverages, and gulping foods and liquids. Diaphragmatic breathing has been demonstrated to be an effective treatment and has become the treatment of choice in this patient population [4]. In patients with underlying depression or anxiety, treatment should include psychological intervention [5]. Patients with co-existing acid reflux may require acid suppressive therapy for management of GERD. When the above treatment approaches have been unsuccessful, baclofen (10 mg three times daily) can be used [6].

References

1. Bredenoord AJ, Weusten BL, Sifrim D, Timmer R, Smout AJ. Aerophagia, gastric, and supragastric belching: a study using intraluminal electrical impedance monitoring. Gut. 2004;53(11):1561.
2. Bredenoord AJ, Smout AJ. Physiologic and pathologic belching. Clin Gastroenterol Hepatol. 2007;5(7):772.
3. Stanghellini V, Chan FK, Hasler WL, Malagelada JR, Suzuki H, Tack J, Talley NJ. Gastroduodenal disorders. Gastroenterology. 2016;150(6):1380–92.
4. Ong AM, Chua LT, Khor CJ, Asokkumar R, Wang YT. Diaphragmatic breathing reduces belching and proton pump inhibitor refractory gastroesophageal reflux symptoms. Clin Gastroenterol Hepatol. 2018;16(3):407–416.e2.
5. Disney B, Trudgill N. Managing a patient with excessive belching. Frontline Gastroenterol. 2014;5(2):79. Epub 2013 Aug 2.
6. Blondeau K, Boecxstaens V, Rommel N, FarréR DS, Holvoet L, Boeckxstaens G, Tack JF. Baclofen improves symptoms and reduces postprandial flow events in patients with rumination and supragastric belching. Clin Gastroenterol Hepatol. 2012;10(4):379–84. Epub 2011 Nov 9.

From Hypercontractile Esophagus to Achalasia

Fahmi Shibli

1   Case Presentation

A 66-year-old woman with a history of atrial fibrillation, hypertension, gastritis, and hypothyroidism presented to our clinic with progressive dysphagia to solids and liquids for over 18 months. She noted the sensation of food getting stuck at the level of her sternum. Her symptoms occurred daily and resulted in an 24 lb weight loss over this period of time. She denied heartburn, regurgitation, choking or coughing during eating, chest pain, vomiting, abdominal pain, or change in bowel habits. Her medications included levothyroxine, metoprolol, pantoprazole, and warfarin. At the time of symptom onset, she underwent a barium swallow, upper endoscopy, and conventional manometry. The barium swallow showed a mildly dilated esophagus with tertiary contractions, delayed emptying of the esophagus, and a narrowed gastroesophageal junction. The upper endoscopy demonstrated normal-appearing esophageal mucosa but with some tightness of the gastroesophageal junction noted (Fig. 1). The patient then underwent conventional manometry which was consistent with a nonspecific esophageal motility disorder. After being lost to follow-up for 1 year, she returned to clinic with the same symptoms, and a high-resolution esophageal manometry (HREM) was performed. This showed a normal median integrated residual pressure (IRP) of 8 mmHg, normal mean resting lower esophageal sphincter (LES) pressure of 21 mmHg, and 30% hypercontractile swallows (Fig. 2). She was diagnosed with hypercontractile esophagus and treated with aggressive acid suppression. Unfortunately, she returned 1 year later without any improvement. She continued to have worsening dysphagia, lost an additional 15 lbs, and reported a new onset of occasional post-prandial chest tightness. A timed barium esophagogram was performed. This study demonstrated diffuse esophageal dilatation with retained secretions and barium with only 20% change in esophageal fluid column

F. Shibli (✉)
Gastroenterology and Liver Diseases, Emek Medical Center, Afula, Israel

© The Author(s), under exclusive license to Springer Nature
Switzerland AG 2024
R. Fass et al. (eds.), *Esophageal Disorders*,
https://doi.org/10.1007/978-3-031-56441-3_11

41

Fig. 1 Normal upper EGD
but with some tightness at
the gastroesophageal
junction

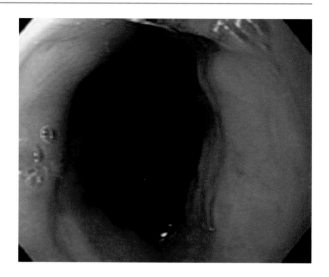

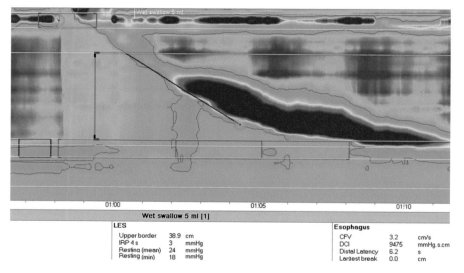

LES			Esophagus		
Upper border	38.9	cm	CFV	3.2	cm/s
IRP 4 s	3	mmHg	DCI	9475	mmHg.s.cm
Resting (mean)	24	mmHg	Distal Latency	6.2	s
Resting (min)	18	mmHg	Largest break	0.0	cm

Fig. 2 A representative swallow from high-resolution esophageal manometry showing a hyper-contractile swallow

after 5 min. In addition, tertiary peristaltic waves within the distal esophagus, limited emptying of the contrast into the stomach, and an air-fluid level were also noted. A repeat HREM was performed (Fig. 3) revealing a markedly elevated IRP and resting LES pressure. There was panesophageal pressurization with every swallow consistent with type II achalasia. The patient underwent Heller myotomy with Dor fundoplication and was subsequently able to tolerate oral intake.

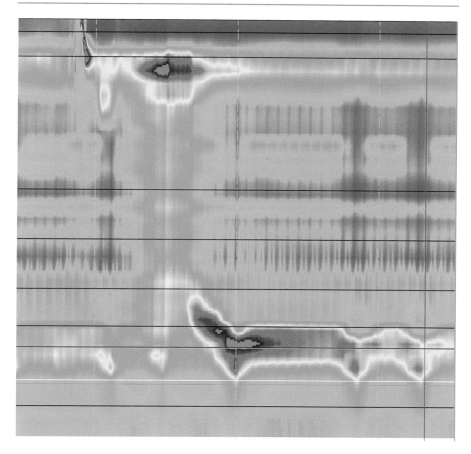

Fig. 3 Representative swallow from repeat high-resolution esophageal manometry showing a lack of relaxation of the lower esophageal sphincter and pan-pressurization of the esophagus

2 Discussion

Here we describe the progression of hypercontractile esophagus to achalasia over a period of about 1 year. Although this is a rare phenomenon, it has been described in the literature [1–11]. Symptoms, especially of dysphagia and weight loss, that seem out of proportion to the manometric diagnosis can prompt a repeat HREM to assess for possible change in diagnosis including progression to achalasia, as was found in this patient. The underlying mechanism behind this progression is still unknown. However, once the progression has occurred, the achalasia is treated as any other achalasia, with myotomy (surgical or endoscopic) or pneumatic dilation. Further research is required to definitively determine whether management strategies should be adjusted for this population.

References

1. Smart HL, Mayberry JF, Atkinson M. Achalasia following gastro-oesophageal reflux. J R Soc Med. 1986;79(2):71–3.
2. Robson K, Rosenberg S, Lembo T. GERD progressing to diffuse esophageal spasm and then to achalasia. Dig Dis Sci. 2000;45(1):110–3.
3. Millan MS, Bourdages R, Beck IT, DaCosta LR. Transition from diffuse esophageal spasm to achalasia. J Clin Gastroenterol. 1979;1(2):107–17.
4. Longstreth GF, Foroozan P. Evolution of symptomatic diffuse esophageal spasm to achalasia. South Med J. 1982;75(2):217–20.
5. Usai Satta P, Oppia F, Piras R, Loriga F. Extrinsic autonomic neuropathy in a case of transition from diffuse esophageal spasm to achalasia. Clin Auton Res. 2004;14(4):270–2.
6. Khatami SS, Khandwala F, Shay SS, Vaezi MF. Does diffuse esophageal spasm progress to achalasia? A prospective cohort study. Dig Dis Sci. 2005;50(9):1605–10.
7. Fontes LH, Herbella FA, Rodriguez TN, Trivino T, Farah JF. Progression of diffuse esophageal spasm to achalasia: incidence and predictive factors. Dis Esophagus. 2013;26(5):470–4.
8. Anggiansah A, Bright NF, McCullagh M, Owen WJ. Transition from nutcracker esophagus to achalasia. Dig Dis Sci. 1990;35(9):1162–6.
9. Paterson WG, Beck IT, Da Costa LR. Transition from nutcracker esophagus to achalasia. A case report. J Clin Gastroenterol. 1991;13(5):554–8.
10. Vantrappen G, Janssens J, Hellemans J, Coremans G. Achalasia, diffuse esophageal spasm, and related motility disorders. Gastroenterology. 1979;76(3):450–7.
11. Abdallah J, Fass R. Progression of jackhammer esophagus to type II achalasia. J Neurogastroenterol Motil. 2016;22(1):153–6. https://doi.org/10.5056/jnm15162.

Is it Reflux or Forceful Contractions?

Sherif Saleh

1   Case Presentation

A 57-year-old woman with reflux symptoms and anxiety presented to the esophageal clinic with a sensation of food infrequently being stuck in her mid-esophagus over the past 3 months. This occurred almost daily and never occurred with liquids. She also notes chronic heartburn that was ongoing for decades but had worsened over the past year. The heartburn was refractory to PPI twice daily therapy. She denied hoarseness, choking episodes, weight loss, or change in appetite. Her only medication was omeprazole 40 mg twice daily.

An upper endoscopy (EGD) revealed mild gastritis and a large 5 cm sliding hiatal hernia (Fig. 1). The esophagus appeared normal. Given high suspicion for GERD and the patient's unwillingness to hold her omeprazole, pH-impedance testing was performed on twice daily PPI. This demonstrated a 6.2% esophageal acid exposure time, with 31 acid reflux events and 57 non-acid reflux events. As the patient reported dysphagia, a high-resolution esophageal manometry (HREM) was performed, with results shown below (Fig. 2). This revealed 20% hypercontractile swallows, with otherwise normal peristalsis and a normal integrated relaxation pressure (IRP). She was diagnosed with hypercontractile esophagus. Due to the prominence of her reflux symptoms and her large hiatal hernia, she underwent laparoscopic Toupet fundoplication. Her symptoms improved postoperatively.

S. Saleh (✉)
Department of Gastroenterology and Hepatology, Case Western Reserve University School of Medicine, MetroHealth Medical Center, Cleveland, OH, USA
e-mail: ssaleh1@metrohealth.org

© The Author(s), under exclusive license to Springer Nature Switzerland AG 2024
R. Fass et al. (eds.), *Esophageal Disorders*,
https://doi.org/10.1007/978-3-031-56441-3_12

45

Fig. 1 Endoscopic image of a large hiatal hernia in retroflexed view

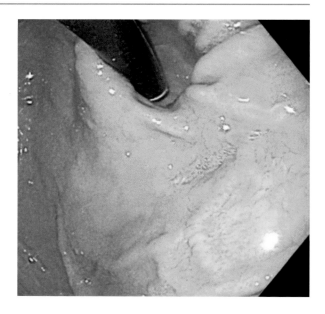

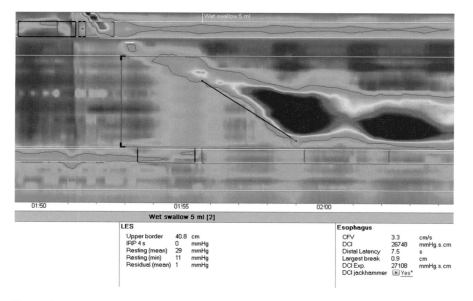

Wet swallow 5 ml [2]						
LES			**Esophagus**			
Upper border	40.8	cm	CFV	3.3	cm/s	
IRP 4 s	0	mmHg	DCI	26748	mmHg.s.cm	
Resting (mean)	29	mmHg	Distal Latency	7.5	s	
Resting (min)	11	mmHg	Largest break	0.9	cm	
Residual (mean)	1	mmHg	DCI Exp.	27108	mmHg.s.cm	
			DCI jackhammer	▶ Yes*		

Fig. 2 A representative swallow from high-resolution esophageal manometry showing a hypercontractile swallow with normal relaxation of the lower esophageal sphincter. Tabular numbers below represent this particular swallow

2   Discussion

This patient presented with worsening dysphagia and reflux symptoms. Her workup revealed both refractory GERD with a large hiatal hernia, as well as hypercontractile esophagus. Management of a patient with both of these diagnoses can be complicated, as antireflux surgery has the potential to exacerbate dysphagia in some patients. However, before developing a management plan for hypercontractile esophagus it is important to search for secondary causes of the disorder. These include uncontrolled GERD, eosinophilic esophagitis, and esophageal outlet obstruction. This patient did have uncontrolled GERD, though it remained unknown whether this was the cause of her hypercontractile esophagus. In the absence of an identifiable secondary cause, hypercontractile esophagus in this patient with only two hypercontractile swallows on manometry and without alarm signs such as weight loss, would be managed conservatively. As there were no plans for invasive management of the hypercontractile esophagus, the patient underwent a partial fundoplication for her refractory GERD. Since both her reflux symptoms and her dysphagia resolved after this procedure, there was no need for further workup or treatment of her hypercontractile esophagus. Had her dysphagia persisted, medical management of hypercontractile esophagus could be considered, including with smooth muscle relaxants such as peppermint oil, calcium channel blockers, tricyclic antidepressants, phosphodiesterase inhibitors or trazodone. Repeat HREM after 6 months could also be considered if the dysphagia did not improve with medical therapy. Should repeat HREM show persistent findings of hypercontractile esophagus that did not respond to medical therapy, endoscopic therapy with Botox injection to the distal esophagus could be considered, though evidence to support its efficacy is limited [1, 2]

Hypercontractile esophagus is defined by abnormally high-amplitude contractions of the esophagus. The pathophysiology of the esophageal contractions in hypercontractile esophagus is thought to be due to excessive cholinergic drive with temporal asynchrony of circular and longitudinal muscle contractions [3]. Typical symptoms are dysphagia, heartburn, and chest pain [4].

Hypercontractile esophagus is diagnosed on HREM when there are at least two liquid swallows with a distal contractile integral (DCI) >8000 mmHg.s.cm with normal relaxation of the esophagogastric junction [5]. Upper endoscopy and barium swallow do not typically show any abnormality.

References

1. Cattau EL Jr, Castell DO, Johnson DA, Spurling TJ, Hirszel R, Chobanian SJ, Richter JE. Diltiazem therapy for symptoms associated with nutcracker esophagus. Am J Gastroenterol. 1991;86(3):272.
2. Cannon RO 3rd, Quyyumi AA, Mincemoyer R, Stine AM, Gracely RH, Smith WB, Geraci MF, Black BC, Uhde TW, Waclawiw MA. Imipramine in patients with chest pain despite normal coronary angiograms. N Engl J Med. 1994;330(20):1411.

3. Jung HY, Puckett JL, Bhalla V, Rojas-Feria M, Bhargava V, Liu J, Mittal RK. Asynchrony between the circular and the longitudinal muscle contraction in patients with nutcracker esophagus. Gastroenterology. 2005;128(5):1179.
4. Herregods TV, Smout AJ, Ooi JL, Sifrim D, Bredenoord AJ. Jackhammer esophagus: observations on a European cohort. Neurogastroenterol Motil. 2017;29(4):e12975. Epub 2016 Oct 17
5. Roman S, Tutuian R. Esophageal hypertensive peristaltic disorders. Neurogastroenterol Motil. 2012;24(Suppl 1):32.

Tasting Acid That Is Not There

Sherif Saleh

1   Case Presentation

A 56-year-old male with a past medical history of hypertension, hyperlipidemia, and a transient ischemic attack presented to the esophageal clinic with 2 years of heartburn, epigastric pain, abdominal bloating, and an acidic taste in his mouth. He also describes overnight frequent regurgitation, especially after eating solid food, which leads to coughing and choking for the last 2 years. He denies chest pain, nausea, vomiting, or any weight loss. He takes tums for abdominal bloating and acidic taste with temporary relief for a few minutes. He does not smoke or drink alcohol regularly. An esophagogastroduodenoscopy (EGD) was performed, which demonstrated mild erythema of the stomach and duodenal bulb but was otherwise normal (Fig. 1). Biopsies ruled out eosinophilic esophagitis (EoE) and *Helicobacter pylori infection*. He was started on a proton pump inhibitor (PPI) twice daily and counseled on lifestyle modifications. Despite optimal therapy, he continued to have epigastric pain and heartburn. The patient underwent wireless esophageal pH testing after stopping his PPI for 2 weeks prior to the procedure. This showed a normal esophageal acid exposure in the supine and upright position with positive symptom indices for heartburn (Fig. 2). He was diagnosed with reflux hypersensitivity and continued on twice daily PPI along with a low-dose tricyclic antidepressant with mild improvement of his symptoms.

S. Saleh (✉)
Department of Gastroenterology and Hepatology, Case Western Reserve University School of Medicine, MetroHealth Medical Center, Cleveland, OH, USA
e-mail: ssaleh1@metrohealth.org

© The Author(s), under exclusive license to Springer Nature Switzerland AG 2024
R. Fass et al. (eds.), *Esophageal Disorders*,
https://doi.org/10.1007/978-3-031-56441-3_13

Fig. 1 Endoscopic image
showing antral erythema

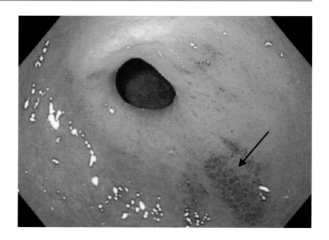

Days	Fraction time pH < 4 (%)		
	Total	Upright	Supine
Day #1	0	0	0
Day #2	0.1	0.2	0
Day #3	1.2	1.4	0
Day #4	0.3	0.3	0.4
Combined	0.4	0.5	0.1

	Heartburn	Chest Pain	Regurgitation
SI:	100	-	-
SAP:	98.1	-	-

Esophageal acid exposure Upright: Normal

Esophageal acid exposure Supine: Normal

Esophageal acid exposure Total: Normal

Fig. 2 Wireless pH testing off of PPI showing normal acid exospore with positive symptom indexes for heartburn consistent with reflux hypersensitivity

2   Discussion

This patient presented with typical GERD symptoms including heartburn and regurgitation, as well as dyspepsia. After an EGD that did not explain the patients symptoms, he was appropriately started on PPI therapy. After escalating to twice daily high dose PPI and still not achieving a satisfactory clinical response, the patient would be classified as having refractory reflux-like symptoms. Patients without proven GERD and with refractory reflux-like symptoms should stop their PPI and undergo reflux testing, ideally with wireless pH testing, in order to determine whether or not they have GERD. In this case, reflux testing off PPI revealed that the patient did not have GERD but a disorder called reflux hypersensitivity. Reflux hypersensitivity is a functional esophageal disorder recognized for the first time by Rome IV criteria, with heartburn being the predominant symptom [1, 2]. It is characterized by a positive association between the predominant symptom and reflux events but in the absence of a pathologic amount of esophageal acid exposure. The diagnosis can be made in a patient with suggestive symptoms and positive association with reflux events based on symptom association probability (SAP) and/or the symptom index (SI). It would be reasonable for a patient such as the one described here to be referred for high-resolution esophageal manometry to rule out a motility disorder prior to confirming the diagnosis of reflux hypersensitivity.

The mechanism of reflux hypersensitivity is thought to be due to esophageal hypersensitivity, which is the perception of non-painful esophageal stimulus as being painful (allodynia) and normally painful esophageal stimulus as being more painful than usual (hyperalgesia) [3].

Management of reflux hypersensitivity can depend on the type of reflux event to which the patient is hypersensitive. The patient in this case was hypersensitive to acid reflux events, and therefore his treatment included maximizing acid suppression. Although not used in our patient, use of histamine-2 receptor antagonists has been shown to reduce esophageal chemoreceptor sensitivity to acid, and these can be used as monotherapy or as an adjunct to PPI [4]. Beyond this, treatment often includes neuromodulation, as was trialed in our patient [1, 5]. There is also some evidence to support the use of acupuncture and hypnotherapy [6]. In our case, the combination of a PPI and a neuromodulator improved the patient's symptoms.

References

1. Yamasaki T, Fass R. Reflux hypersensitivity: a new functional esophageal disorder. J Neurogastroenterol Motil. 2017;23(4):495–503.
2. Aziz Q, Fass R, Gyawali CP, Miwa H, Pandolfino JE, Zerbib F. Esophageal disorders. Gastroenterology. 2016;150:1368–79.
3. Dickman R, Maradey-Romero C, Fass R. The role of pain modulators in esophageal disorders - no pain no gain. Neurogastroenterol Motil. 2014;26:603–10.
4. Marrero JM, de Caestecker JS, Maxwell JD. Effect of famotidine on oesophageal sensitivity in gastro-oesophageal reflux disease. Gut. 1994;35:447–50.
5. Gyawali CP, Fass R. Management of gastroesophageal reflux disease. Gastroenterology. 2018;154(2):302–18.
6. Dickman R, Schiff E, Holland A, Wright C, Sarela SR, Han B, Fass R. Clinical trial: acupuncture vs. doubling the proton pump inhibitor dose in refractory heartburn. Aliment Pharmacol Ther. 2007;26(10):1333–44.

Disorder of Esophageal Motility After Chemotherapy and Radiation

Yeseong Kim

1 Case Presentation

A 61-year-old female with atrial fibrillation, congestive heart failure, hypertension, and breast cancer presented to the gastroenterology clinic with a chief complaint of difficulty swallowing. The patient noted that both solid and liquid foods would become stuck in the middle of her chest, resulting in dull pain. These episodes lasted up to 1 min and were usually relieved by drinking sips of water. Swallowing was not painful in itself and did not result in coughing, choking, or nasal regurgitation. She had no weight loss or change in appetite and no nausea, vomiting, abdominal pain, or heartburn. Ten years prior to her current presentation, the patient received adjuvant chemotherapy and radiotherapy following mastectomy for her breast cancer.

Her symptoms and history were concerning for an esophageal anatomical cause for her dysphagia, and she was referred for esophagogastroduodenoscopy (EGD) with biopsies. EGD revealed a partial non-obstructing Schatzki's ring at the distal esophagus (Fig. 1) but was otherwise unremarkable. The esophageal ring was not believed to be narrow enough to cause the patient's dysphagia. Biopsies were negative for eosinophilic esophagitis. Subsequently, the patient underwent high-resolution esophageal manometry (HREM), which revealed normal peristalsis with an elevated integrated relaxation pressure (IRP) on supine and upright positions, suggestive of a diagnosis of esophagogastric junction outflow obstruction (EGJOO) (Fig. 2). Following the diagnosis, computed tomography (CT) of the chest and abdomen was obtained to evaluate for extra-esophageal etiologies of EGJ outflow obstruction, which revealed a small hiatal hernia (Fig. 3). The patient was managed conservatively by lifestyle modifications, but her symptoms persisted.

Y. Kim (✉)
Division of Gastroenterology and Hepatology, Lewis Katz School of Medicine at Temple University, Temple University Hospital, Philadelphia, PA, USA

© The Author(s), under exclusive license to Springer Nature Switzerland AG 2024
R. Fass et al. (eds.), *Esophageal Disorders*,
https://doi.org/10.1007/978-3-031-56441-3_14

Fig. 1 EGD
demonstrating a partial
non-obstructing Schatzki's
ring at the distal esophagus
but without additional
pathology

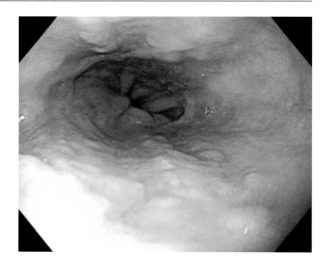

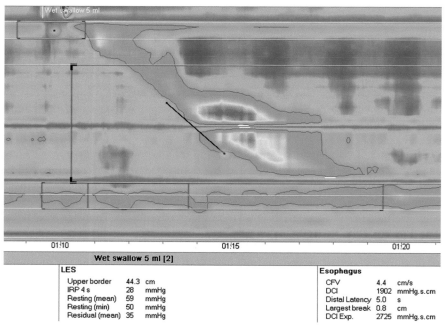

LES			Esophagus		
Upper border	44.3	cm	CFV	4.4	cm/s
IRP 4 s	28	mmHg	DCI	1902	mmHg.s.cm
Resting (mean)	59	mmHg	Distal Latency	5.0	s
Resting (min)	50	mmHg	Largest break	0.8	cm
Residual (mean)	35	mmHg	DCI Exp.	2725	mmHg.s.cm

Fig. 2 Representative swallow from high-resolution esophageal manometry revealing an elevated integrated relaxation pressure with normal peristalsis

Fig. 3 CT scan showing a small hiatal hernia with no external compression of the esophagus

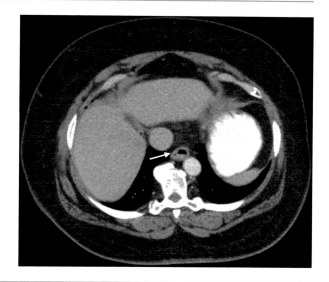

2   Discussion

This case describes a patient with dysphagia diagnosed with EGJOO based on her HREM findings of high IRP in supine and upright position with no etiologies of outflow obstruction noted on imaging [1]. It is unclear whether the prior chemotherapy or radiotherapy caused her dysphagia symptoms or contributed to her EGJOO diagnosis. Common esophageal complications post-radiotherapy typically include esophagitis and strictures, but there have also been some reports of radiation-induced esophageal motor dysfunction [2, 3]. However, there is currently no data on EGJOO diagnosis after radiotherapy or systemic chemotherapy. Other potential secondary causes of EGJOO, such as opiate use and external compression from a large hiatal or paraesophageal hernia, were ruled out in our patient by medication history and CT of the chest. The non-obstructing Schatzki's ring and small hiatal hernia were not significant enough to be the cause of the outlet obstruction. Endoscopic ultrasound of the EGJ can be another useful modality in this regard.

Given the mild to moderate nature of our patient's symptoms, initial management was conservative, with dysphagia precautions and observation. However, our patient's symptoms persisted despite this. Appropriate next steps in management would include repeating HREM 6 months later to confirm the diagnostic criteria are still met and timed barium esophagram to determine severity of the obstruction with a 13 mm barium tablet to asses for a more subtle transient obstruction in the passage of solid boluses. Pharmacologic therapy including calcium channel blockers such as diltiazem or acetylcholinesterase inhibitors such as acetamide may be considered but do not have a high rate of efficacy [4, 5].

References

1. Yadlapati R, Kahrilas PJ, Fox MR, Bredenoord AJ, et al. Esophageal motility disorders on high-resolution manometry: Chicago classification version 4.0©. Neurogastroenterol Motil. 2021;33(1):e14058.
2. Vitton V, Andrianjafy C, Luciano L, Gonzalez JM, Padovani L. Radio-induced esophageal motility disorders: an unrecognized diagnosis. Cancer Radiother. 2021;25(3):249–53.
3. Seeman H, Gates JA, Traube M. Esophageal motor dysfunction years after radiation therapy. Dig Dis Sci. 1992;37(2):303–6.
4. Pérez-Fernández MT, Santander C, Marinero A, Burgos-Santamaría D, Chavarría-Herbozo C. Characterization and follow-up of esophagogastric junction outflow obstruction detected by high resolution manometry. Neurogastroenterol Motil. 2016;28(1):116–26.
5. Van Hoeij F, Smout A, Bredenoord A. Characterization of idiopathic esophagogastric junction outflow obstruction. Neurogastroenterol Motil. 2015;27(9):1310–6.

Achalasia Masquerading as Reflux

Yeseong Kim

1 Case Presentation

A 71-year-old female with hypertension, chronic kidney disease, coronary artery disease, myocardial infarction, and prior omental infarction, presented to the gastroenterology clinic for 2 years of reflux symptoms. She described burning, retrosternal pain associated with a sour taste in her mouth. Her symptoms arose primarily following eating spicy or acidic foods such as tomato sauces and chili peppers. This sensation of burning in her throat caused recurrent episodes of nausea resulting in intermittent vomiting. She denied symptoms of dysphagia, odynophagia, anorexia, weight loss, melena, or hematochezia. The patient underwent computed tomography (CT) of the abdomen for unrelated abdominal pain which incidentally identified a severely dilated and fluid-filled esophagus with a sharp transition at the esophagogastric junction (EGJ) (Fig. 1). The patient underwent esophagogastroduodenoscopy (EGD) which revealed a diffusely dilated and tortuous esophagus and a tight EGJ (Fig. 2). Esophageal biopsies showed evidence of reflux disease with no evidence of eosinophilic esophagitis. She was then referred for a timed barium esophagram, which showed a dilated and sigmoid-shaped esophagus with moderate retention of barium at the distal esophagus unchanged between 0- and 5-min images. A high-resolution esophageal manometry (HREM) was then performed, revealing absent peristalsis with 50% of swallows showing pan-pressurization of the esophagus (Fig. 3). The catheter did not cross the EGJ, and thus the IRP could not be manometrically evaluated. However, based on the findings in the body of the esophagus combined with the results of the barium esophagram and EGD findings, the patient was diagnosed with type II achalasia. She underwent peroral endoscopic myotomy (POEM) with improvement in her symptoms.

Y. Kim (✉)
Division of Gastroenterology and Hepatology, Lewis Katz School of Medicine at Temple University, Temple University Hospital, Philadelphia, PA, USA

© The Author(s), under exclusive license to Springer Nature Switzerland AG 2024
R. Fass et al. (eds.), *Esophageal Disorders*,
https://doi.org/10.1007/978-3-031-56441-3_15

57

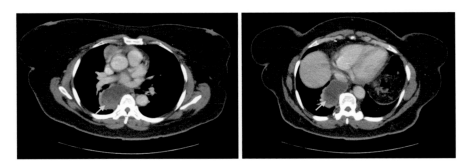

Fig. 1 CT with contrast showing severely dilated distal esophagus with fluid

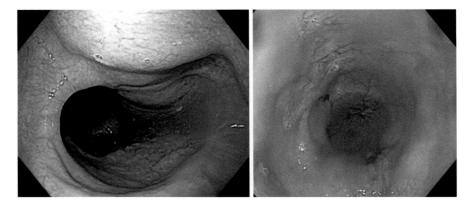

Fig. 2 EGD showing a dilated and tortuous esophagus with a tight EGJ

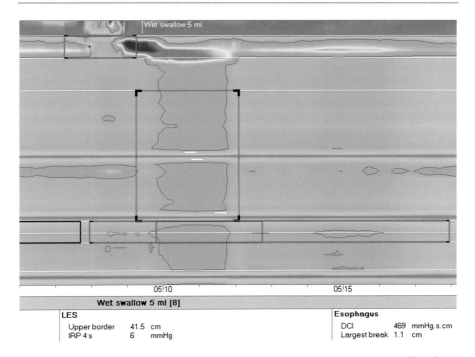

LES			Esophagus		
Upper border	41.5	cm	DCI	469	mmHg.s.cm
IRP 4 s	6	mmHg	Largest break	1.1	cm

Fig. 3 A representative swallow from high-resolution esophageal manometry revealing absent peristalsis with pan-pressurization of the esophagus and elevated integrated relaxation pressure tabular numbers pertain to this particular swallow

2 Discussion

Achalasia is defined by lack of incomplete lower esophageal sphincter (LES) relaxation in the setting of absent esophageal peristalsis [1, 2]. There are three subtypes of achalasia, differentiated by the pattern of non-peristaltic esophageal pressurization that can be seen on HREM [2]. Our patient was diagnosed with type II achalasia, which is defined by Chicago 4.0 as an abnormal median IRP and absent contractility (100% failed peristalsis) with panesophageal pressurization in 20% or more swallows [2]. The classic presentation of achalasia is progressive dysphagia to both solids and liquids (>90%), though other symptoms such as heartburn, epigastric pain, regurgitation, and cough occur frequently (>20%) [3]. It is important to note that not all patients with achalasia will report dysphagia. This case provides a unique example of a patient eventually diagnosed with type II achalasia who initially presented with reflux symptoms and without symptoms of dysphagia to either solids or liquids. Reflux symptoms likely occurred in this patient due to the retention of food and pills in the esophagus, with regurgitation.

Between the three subtypes of achalasia, type II carries the most favorable prognosis, with a 96% success rate in treatment with either Heller myotomy, POEM or pneumatic dilation [4]. Our patient had improvement in her reported symptoms postoperatively.

References

1. Pandolfino JE, Gawron AJ. Achalasia: a systematic review. JAMA. 2015;313(18):1841–52.
2. Yadlapati R, Kahrilas PJ, Fox MR, et al. Esophageal motility disorders on high-resolution manometry: Chicago classification version 4.0©. Neurogastroenterol Motil. 2021;33(1):e14058.
3. Tsuboi K, Hoshino M, Srinivasan A, Yano F, Hinder RA, DeMeester TR, et al. Insights gained from symptom evaluation of esophageal motility disorders: a review of 4,215 patients. Digestion. 2012;85(3):236–42.
4. Rohof WO, Salvador R, Annese V, des Varannes SB, Chaussade S, Costantini M, et al. Outcomes of treatment for achalasia depend on manometric subtype. Gastroenterology. 2013;144(4):718–25.

Progression of Distal Esophageal Spasm to Achalasia

Yeseong Kim

1   Case Presentation

A 40-year-old female with a past medical history of thyroid goiter and chronic reflux symptoms presented to the gastroenterology clinic with difficulty swallowing. At the time of the initial encounter, the patient reported that she had been experiencing symptoms during swallows for approximately 10 months that were increasing in frequency. Her symptoms consisted of a sticking sensation in the back of her throat when trying to swallow either solid or liquid foods. She further reported ongoing acid reflux symptoms which were usually relieved by taking over-the-counter antacids or ginger ale. Sitting up straight and waiting for the episodes to pass also helped mitigate her symptoms. She denied symptoms of choking, coughing, or nasal regurgitation during swallows. She also did not have any nausea, vomiting, anorexia, weight loss, or abdominal pain. A barium esophagram was performed and showed air-fluid level at the distal esophagus, a nonspecific peristaltic abnormality, and delayed passage of a barium tablet (Fig. 1). The patient was sent for an esophagogastroduodenoscopy (EGD), which revealed mild antral gastritis but normal esophageal mucosa and biopsies negative for eosinophilic esophagitis. The patient was then referred for high-resolution esophageal manometry (HREM), which showed a normal integrated relaxation pressure (IRP) and 70% premature contractions, consistent with a diagnosis of distal esophageal spasm (DES). Following diagnosis, the patient was started on diltiazem 60 mg four times a day and instructed to continue her proton pump inhibitor. The patient returned to the GI clinic several months later, reporting improved dysphagia symptoms but increased headaches and dizziness as side effects from the diltiazem. Her dose was reduced at the time, which led to a return of her dysphagia symptoms. Her regimen was

Y. Kim (✉)
Division of Gastroenterology and Hepatology, Lewis Katz School of Medicine at Temple University, Temple University Hospital, Philadelphia, PA, USA

© The Author(s), under exclusive license to Springer Nature Switzerland AG 2024
R. Fass et al. (eds.), *Esophageal Disorders*,
https://doi.org/10.1007/978-3-031-56441-3_16

Fig. 1 Barium swallow
showing air-fluid levels at
the distal esophagus

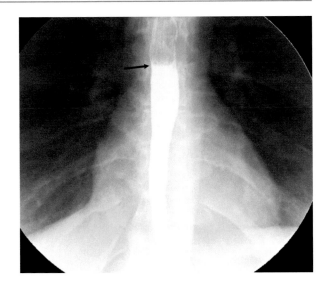

Fig. 2 EGD with mild
resistance when advancing
the scope through the LES
but with no esophageal
obstruction that could be
visualized throughout the
esophagus

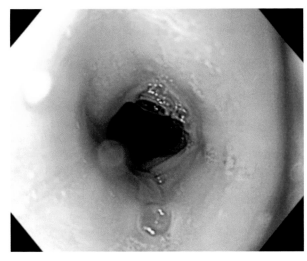

eventually switched to the long-acting formulation of diltiazem at 180 mg daily, which controlled her symptoms well without side effects. Several years later, the patient returned to the GI clinic reporting intermittent return of dysphagia symptoms, for which she was started on imipramine 50 mg as needed during breakthrough episodes. However, she continued to report intermittent symptoms of dysphagia. Repeat EGD was done, which revealed a new finding of increased resistance during passage of the endoscope through the lower esophageal sphincter (LES) without obvious anatomical abnormality (Fig. 2), concerning for a new esophageal motility disorder. She was referred to repeat HREM, which showed an

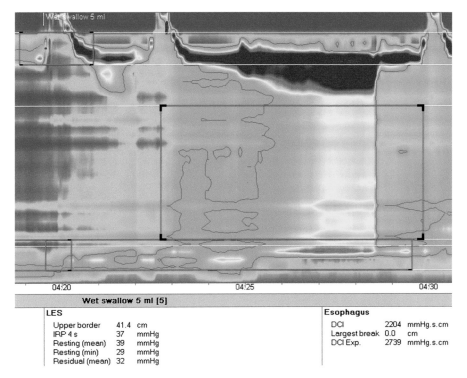

Fig. 3 A representative swallow from high-resolution esophageal manometry showing an elevated integrated relaxation pressure and pan-pressurization of the esophagus

elevated IRP of 29.55 mmHg and 100% pan-pressurization of the esophagus (Fig. 3). She was diagnosed with type II achalasia and referred for peroral endoscopic myotomy (POEM) with resolution of her symptoms.

2 Discussion

This is a unique case of DES that later progressed to type II achalasia [1]. The progression of DES to achalasia is an uncommon phenomenon and has been reported in the literature with an incidence rate ranging between 8 to 14% in adults [2, 3]. In a prospective study of 73 patients, dysphagia and distal simultaneous waves with low amplitude were identified as potential risk factors of disease progression from DES to achalasia. The authors recommended that patients with these risk factors undergo repeat manometry after 2 years of diagnosis of DES [3].

The mechanism of progression from DES to achalasia and what triggers it remain unknown. However, identifying progression of DES to achalasia is particularly important as the management does change and patients with achalasia have a more predictable and favorable outcome after invasive therapeutic procedures compared to patients with DES. Management of patients with DES that progressed to achalasia is currently the same as for all patients with achalasia. Further research is needed to determine whether this patient population would benefit from different management strategies.

References

1. Yadlapati R, Pandolfino JE, Fox MR, Bredenoord AJ, Kahrilas PJ. What is new in Chicago classification version 4.0? Neurogastroenterol Motil. 2021;33(1):e14053.
2. Khatami SS, Khandwala F, Shay SS, Vaezi MF. Does diffuse esophageal spasm progress to achalasia? A prospective cohort study. Dig Dis Sci. 2005;50(9):1605–10.
3. Fontes LH, Herbella FA, Rodriguez TN, Trivino T, Farah JF. Progression of diffuse esophageal spasm to achalasia: incidence and predictive factors. Dis Esophagus. 2013;26(5):470–4. https://doi.org/10.1111/j.1442-2050.2012.01377.x. Epub 2012 Jul 20.

Dysphagia to Solids and Liquids

Yeseong Kim

1   Case Presentation

A 74-year-old male with aortic valve stenosis, hypertension, hyperlipidemia, previous duodenal ulcer, iron deficiency anemia, and decompensated alcoholic liver cirrhosis with ascites presented to the gastroenterology clinic with dysphagia. He reported that his dysphagia occurred about twice per week for both solids and liquids, and it felt like foods were getting stuck in his lower throat. He denied weight loss or anorexia, bloody or black stools, recurrent nausea or vomiting, or abdominal pain. He had undergone multiple esophagogastroduodenoscopies (EGDs) which were unremarkable (Fig. 1). His reflux symptoms were well controlled on omeprazole 20 mg daily. He was referred for high-resolution esophageal manometry (HREM), which revealed an abnormally high integrated relaxation pressure (IRP) of 23 mmHg, a high mean resting lower esophageal sphincter (LES) pressure of 70 mmHg, and 100% pan-pressurization of the esophagus consistent with type II achalasia (Fig. 2). A timed barium esophagram showed significant delay in esophageal emptying with retained contrast to the level of the thoracic inlet at 1-, 2-, and 5-min images with little interval change in the intraesophageal contrast volume between 0 and 5 min. The esophagram also revealed a dilated proximal esophagus, tortuous distal esophagus with narrowed esophagogastric junction, and tertiary contractions throughout the intrathoracic esophagus (Fig. 3). He was initially planned for an EGD with botulinum toxin injection, but this was ultimately deferred after he was discovered to have advanced colon cancer.

Y. Kim (✉)
Division of Gastroenterology and Hepatology, Lewis Katz School of Medicine at Temple University, Temple University Hospital, Philadelphia, PA, USA

© The Author(s), under exclusive license to Springer Nature Switzerland AG 2024
R. Fass et al. (eds.), *Esophageal Disorders*,
https://doi.org/10.1007/978-3-031-56441-3_17

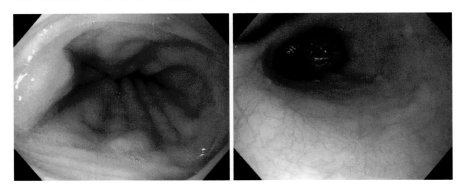

Fig. 1 Unremarkable EGD

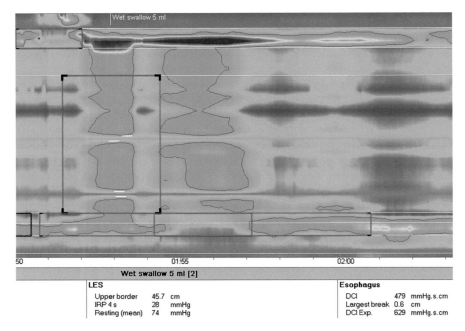

LES			Esophagus		
Upper border	45.7	cm	DCI	479	mmHg.s.cm
IRP 4 s	28	mmHg	Largest break	0.6	cm
Resting (mean)	74	mmHg	DCI Exp.	629	mmHg.s.cm

Fig. 2 Representative swallow from high-resolution esophageal manometry revealing an abnormally high integrated relaxation pressure and pan-pressurization of the esophagus

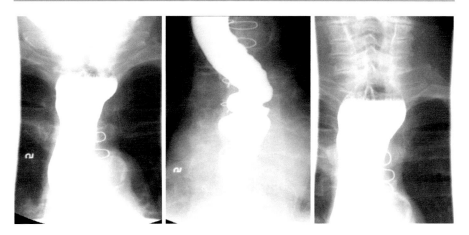

Fig. 3 Esophagram showing a dilated proximal esophagus, tortuous distal esophagus with narrowed esophagogastric junction, and tertiary contractions throughout the intrathoracic esophagus

2 Discussion

Achalasia is an esophageal motility disorder thought to be caused by degeneration of the myenteric plexus and vagus nerve fibers innervating the lower esophageal sphincter (LES), leading to incomplete LES relaxation in the setting of absent esophageal peristalsis [1]. There are three subtypes of achalasia, differentiated by the pattern of non-peristaltic esophageal pressurization that can be seen on HREM [2]. Type II achalasia, which is the diagnosis in this patient, is defined by an abnormal median IRP and absent contractility (100% failed peristalsis) with panesophageal pressurization in 20% or more swallows [2].

The most common symptom of achalasia is dysphagia, and it often occurs with both solid and liquid intake [3]. It is important to note that the location of the obstruction experienced by the patient does not necessarily correlate with the primary anatomic location of the pathology. In our case, the patient experienced food sticking in his throat. This should not preclude achalasia, in which the primary obstruction occurs at the LES.

Diagnosis of achalasia requires first ruling out mechanical obstruction by EGD, followed by HREM [4]. Timed barium esophagram and EndoFlip are useful tests to diagnose and monitor therapeutic interventions in patients with achalasia [5].

References

1. Pandolfino JE, Gawron AJ. Achalasia: a systematic review. JAMA. 2015;313(18):1841–52.
2. Yadlapati R, Kahrilas PJ, Fox MR, et al. Esophageal motility disorders on high-resolution manometry: Chicago classification version 4.0©. Neurogastroenterol Motil. 2021;33(1):e14058.

3. Tsuboi K, Hoshino M, Srinivasan A, Yano F, Hinder RA, DeMeester TR, et al. Insights gained from symptom evaluation of esophageal motility disorders: a review of 4,215 patients. Digestion. 2012;85(3):236–42.
4. Pandolfino JE, Kwiatek MA, Nealis T, Bulsiewicz W, Post J, Kahrilas PJ. Achalasia: a new clinically relevant classification by high-resolution manometry. Gastroenterology. 2008;135(5):1526–33.
5. Neyaz Z, Gupta M, Ghoshal UC. How to perform and interpret timed barium esophagogram. J Neurogastroenterol Motil. 2013;19(2):251–6.

Progressive Intermittent Dysphagia

Sara Ghoneim

1   Case Presentation

A 54-year-old male was seen in the gastroenterology clinic with a 10-year history of progressive intermittent dysphagia to solids and liquids associated with heartburn. Previous endoscopy had shown LA grade A reflux esophagitis and erosive gastropathy. He was started on once daily proton pump inhibitor (PPI) without much relief, and he returned to the clinic with persistent symptoms. A repeat upper endoscopy revealed healing of his erosive esophagitis and a small mid-esophageal erosion (Fig. 1). Biopsies were negative for eosinophilic esophagitis. He subsequently underwent high-resolution esophageal manometry (HREM), which showed a normal median integrated relaxation pressure (IRP) and lower esophageal sphincter (LES) resting pressure, 10% normal swallows, 40% failed swallows, and 50% simultaneous contractions of the distal esophagus (Fig. 2). The patient was diagnosed with distal esophageal spasm (DES) and was started on twice daily PPI. Unfortunately, the patient was subsequently lost to follow-up.

S. Ghoneim (✉)
Department of Gastroenterology and Hepatology, University of Nebraska College of Medicine, University of Nebraska Medical Center, Omaha, NE, USA

© The Author(s), under exclusive license to Springer Nature Switzerland AG 2024
R. Fass et al. (eds.), *Esophageal Disorders*,
https://doi.org/10.1007/978-3-031-56441-3_18

Fig. 1 The upper
endoscopy was
unremarkable

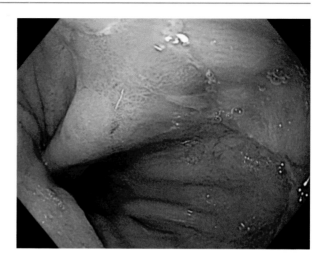

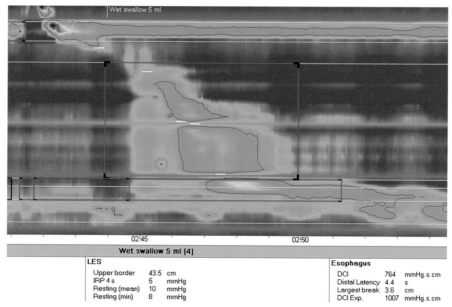

LES				Esophagus		
Upper border	43.5	cm		DCI	764	mmHg.s.cm
IRP 4 s	5	mmHg		Distal Latency	4.4	s
Resting (mean)	10	mmHg		Largest break	3.6	cm
Resting (min)	8	mmHg		DCI Exp.	1007	mmHg.s.cm

Fig. 2 Representative swallow from high-resolution esophageal manometry demonstrating a normal median integrated relaxation pressure, with a simultaneous contraction of the distal esophagus. Tabular numbers below represent this particular swallow

2   Discussion

DES is a disorder of peristalsis defined by premature contractions in at least 20% of swallows with a normal IRP [1]. Patients with DES generally present with dysphagia, as well as retrosternal chest pain. It is thought that dysphagia occurs because the disordered peristalsis does not advance the food bolus into the stomach. [2]. Radiographic findings of DES classically display a "corkscrew" esophagus, though in practice this finding is relatively rare, and most barium esophagrams will show non-specific findings [2].

According to one study, only 2% of patients presenting with dysphagia and chest pain have DES [3]. It is thought that DES occurs due to impaired esophageal inhibitory innervation resulting in premature and rapid contractions in the distal esophagus [4].

Excessive acetylcholine release or insufficient nitric oxide may contribute to the development of DES [5]. Diagnosis of DES requires the exclusion of secondary causes of simultaneous contractions of the esophagus such as gastroesophageal reflux disease, obstruction of the distal esophagus, and opiate use.

There is a lack of high-quality data to support any particular treatment modality for DES. Typically, treatment begins by optimizing gastroesophageal reflux therapy in patients with GERD, as was attempted in this patient [6]. Additionally, pharmacologic therapies include smooth muscle relaxants such as calcium channel blockers, nitrates, or peppermint oil, though there is limited data to support their efficacy. Neuromodulation with low-dose tricyclic anti-depressants has also been used. Patients who do not respond to pharmacologic therapy can be considered for invasive approaches including botulinum toxin injections to the distal esophagus, peroral endoscopic myotomy, and long Heller myotomy. However, these interventions lack high-quality efficacy data to support their routine use [7].

References

1. Schlottmann F, Herbella FA, Patti MG. Understanding the Chicago classification: from tracings to patients. J Neurogastroenterol Motil. 2017;23(4):487–94. https://doi.org/10.5056/jnm17026.
2. Khalaf M, Chowdhary S, Elias PS, Castell D. Distal esophageal spasm: a review. Am J Med. 2018;131(9):1034–40. https://doi.org/10.1016/j.amjmed.2018.02.031.
3. Pandolfino JE, et al. Distal esophageal spasm in high-resolution esophageal pressure topography: defining clinical phenotypes. Gastroenterology. 2011;141(2):469–75. https://doi.org/10.1053/j.gastro.2011.04.058.
4. Rohof WOA, Bredenoord AJ. Chicago classification of esophageal motility disorders: lessons learned. Curr Gastroenterol Rep. 2017;19(8):37. https://doi.org/10.1007/s11894-017-0576-7.
5. Valdovinos MA, Zavala-Solares MR, Coss-Adame E. Esophageal hypomotility and spastic motor disorders: current diagnosis and treatment. Curr Gastroenterol Rep. 2014;16(11):421.
6. Achem SR, Gerson LB. Distal esophageal spasm: an update. Curr Gastroenterol Rep. 2013;15(9):325.
7. Khashab MA, Benias PC, Swanstrom LL. Endoscopic Myotomy for foregut motility disorders. Gastroenterology. 2018;154(7):1901–10.

A Post-Fundoplication Surprise

Sara Ghoneim

1   Case Presentation

A 65-year-old African American male was referred to the gastroenterology clinic for frequent hiccups and heartburn. His medical history included well-controlled type 2 diabetes, hypertension, hyperlipidemia, and Chiari-I malformation with hydromyelia in the cervical cord. His symptoms began at age 50 when he complained of frequent hiccups, bland regurgitation, and heartburn that did not respond to proton pump inhibitor treatment. A previous upper endoscopy revealed a mildly tortuous esophagus with a 4–5 cm hiatal hernia and Cameron erosions. Ultimately, he underwent laparoscopic Nissen fundoplication with hiatal hernia repair. Unfortunately, after the surgery he continued to have constant belching and bland regurgitation. Six months after surgery, he underwent a timed barium esophagogram which was notable for a dilated esophagus with severe esophageal dysmotility evidenced by retained contrast to the level of mid intrathoracic esophagus at 5 minutes (Fig. 1). This study also revealed a slipped Nissen with migration of the wrap proximally above the level of the diaphragm and mechanical obstruction of the distal esophagus. He subsequently underwent an upper endoscopy which showed a large diaphragmatic hernia along with severe LA Grade C erosive esophagitis, a dilated and tortuous esophagus (Fig. 2). High-resolution esophageal manometry (HREM) was performed and showed high median integrated resting pressure (IRP) and 100% failed peristalsis (Fig. 3). The patient was diagnosed with type I achalasia post-Nissen fundoplication and referred for surgical evaluation for Nissen reversal with myotomy. The patient declined surgical intervention and unfortunately did not return to gastroenterology clinic.

S. Ghoneim (✉)
Department of Gastroenterology and Hepatology, University of Nebraska College of Medicine, University of Nebraska Medical Center, Omaha, NE, USA

© The Author(s), under exclusive license to Springer Nature Switzerland AG 2024
R. Fass et al. (eds.), *Esophageal Disorders*,
https://doi.org/10.1007/978-3-031-56441-3_19

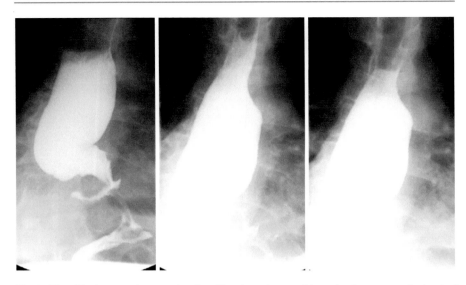

Fig. 1 Timed barium esophagram showing dilated esophagus with retained contrast to the level of mid intrathoracic esophagus at 5 minutes

Fig. 2 EGD showing LA
grade C erosive esophagitis

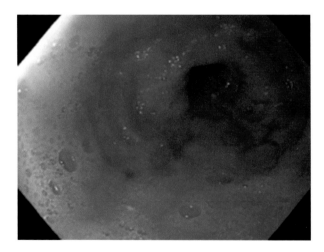

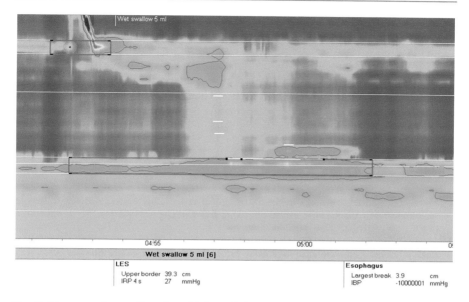

Fig. 3 Representative swallow from high-resolution esophageal manometry showing a failed swallow with high median integrated relaxation pressure. Tabular numbers pertain to this particular swallow

2   Discussion

Laparoscopic Nissen fundoplication serves to restore the integrity of the barrier between the esophagus and stomach in patients with uncontrolled acid reflux [1]. Nonetheless, this procedure is associated with complications in up to 10% of patients, including partial or complete breakdown of the fundoplication with recurrent gastroesophageal reflux, slipped fundoplication, or tight fundoplication resulting in postoperative dysphagia [2]. Dysphagia after fundoplication may persist due to complications of the wrap, a newly diagnosed motility disorder, and a previously unrecognized motility disorder or peptic stricture [3]. It is now standard of care that candidates for antireflux surgery undergo preoperative HREM in order to identify esophageal motility disorders prior to surgical fundoplication. In our case, HREM was not performed in advance of the surgery. Thus, whether the patient had achalasia all along or whether he developed pseudoachalasia due to tight fundoplication remains unknown, though no endoscopic findings suggestive of achalasia were noted in the preoperative EGD.

Patients with dysphagia after fundoplication must undergo investigation to determine the etiology, usually beginning with EGD, but often including timed barium esophagram with a 13 mm barium tablet and HREM. Pseudoachalasia, also referred to as secondary achalasia, after laparoscopic Nissen fundoplication is an uncommon complication in patients with documented normal esophageal motility prior surgery and is attributed to tight surgical fundoplication [4–6].

The pathogenesis of pseudoachalasia after Nissen fundoplication is currently unknown but likely relates to prolonged obstruction of the distal esophagus by the fundoplication wrap, resulting in loss of esophageal peristalsis. Alternatively, vagal nerve injury during surgery or by disruption of the myenteric plexus at the site of fundoplication construction may result in secondary achalasia [4–6]. Although uncommon, 12% of pseudoachalasia cases are due to surgeries involving the esophagus and GE junction, with the remainder being from primary and secondary malignancies [7].

References

1. Morais DJ, Lopes LR, Andreollo NA. Dysphagia after antireflux fundoplication: endoscopic, radiological and manometric evaluation. Arq Bras Cir Dig. 2014;27(4):251–5. https://doi.org/10.1590/S0102-67202014000400006.
2. Hinder RA, Filipi CJ, Wetscher G, Neary P, DeMeester TR, Perdikis G. Laparoscopic Nissen fundoplication is an effective treatment for gastroesophageal reflux disease. Ann Surg. 1994;220(4):472–83. https://doi.org/10.1097/00000658-199410000-00006.
3. Richter J. Gastroesophageal reflux disease treatment: side effects and complications of fundoplication. Clin Gastroenterol Hepatol. 2013;11:465–71.
4. Carlson MA, Frantzides CT. Complications and results of primary minimally invasive antireflux procedures: a review of 10,735 reported cases. J Am Coll Surg. 2001;193:428–39.
5. Stylopoulos N, Bunker CJ, Rttner DW. Development of achalasia secondary to laparoscopic Nissen fundoplication. J Gastrointest Surg. 2002;6:368–76.
6. Harbaugh JW, Clayton SB. Pseudoachalasia following Nissen fundoplication. ACG Case Rep J. 2020;7(2):e00318.
7. Abubakar U, Bashir M, Kesieme E. Pseudoachalasia: A review. Niger J Clin Pract. 2016;19(3):303.

Difficulty Swallowing After Open Heart Surgery

Sara Ghoneim

1 Case Presentation

A 66-year-old male was seen in the gastroenterology clinic for dysphagia that started 1 month after coronary artery bypass graft (CABG). He described a progressive sensation of food getting stuck at the level of his neck, which was occurring daily, but only to solids. He also reported hoarseness and an unintentional weight loss of 10 pounds. He denied chest pain, regurgitation, nausea, or vomiting. Past medical history was significant for obesity, hypertension, poorly controlled type two diabetes, coronary artery disease, and iron deficiency anemia. An upper endoscopy with biopsies was performed and showed a normal esophagus with no explanation for dysphagia. He also underwent a modified barium swallow, which revealed prolonged mastication of solids and mild delayed initiation of pharyngeal swallow with pureed and thin liquids without evidence of aspiration or laryngeal penetration. He started working with speech therapy with improvement in his hoarseness, but his dysphagia worsened and he was unable to swallow pills or liquids, leading to further weight loss and decreased oral intake. He was therefore referred for high-resolution esophageal manometry (HREM), which demonstrated normal median integrated relaxation pressure (IRP) with 30% hypercontractile swallows (Fig. 1). The patient was diagnosed with hypercontractile esophagus but unfortunately was then lost to follow-up.

S. Ghoneim (✉)
Department of Gastroenterology and Hepatology, University of Nebraska College of Medicine, University of Nebraska Medical Center, Omaha, NE, USA

© The Author(s), under exclusive license to Springer Nature Switzerland AG 2024
R. Fass et al. (eds.), *Esophageal Disorders*,
https://doi.org/10.1007/978-3-031-56441-3_20

77

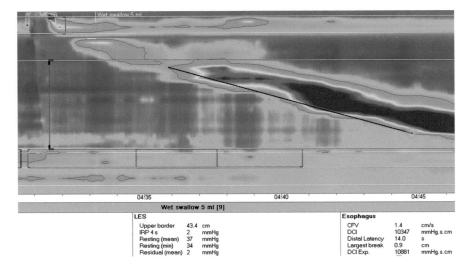

Wet swallow 5 ml [9]					
LES			**Esophagus**		
Upper border	43.4	cm	CFV	1.4	cm/s
IRP 4 s	2	mmHg	DCI	10347	mmHg.s.cm
Resting (mean)	37	mmHg	Distal Latency	14.0	s
Resting (min)	34	mmHg	Largest break	0.9	cm
Residual (mean)	2	mmHg	DCI Exp.	10881	mmHg.s.cm

Fig. 1 Representative swallow from high-resolution esophageal manometry showing a hypercontractile swallow with normal integrated relaxation pressure and a high distal contractile integral. Tabular numbers pertain to this particular swallow

2 Discussion

Our patient presented with dysphagia that began after CABG and was diagnosed with hypercontractile esophagus, a rare esophageal motility disorder characterized by excessively strong peristaltic contractions of the esophagus. Patients typically present with dysphagia, as our patient did, or chest pain.

To our knowledge, this is the first reported case of hypercontractile esophagus after CABG. The patient also experienced hoarseness which is seen postoperatively, in 10–15% of cardiovascular interventions, due to recurrent laryngeal nerve injury [1]. As the vagus nerve or recurrent laryngeal nerve travels in proximity to cardiovascular structures, we hypothesize that our patient might have experienced hypercontractile esophagus due to vagal nerve injury during CABG.

As there are no prospective studies addressing the management of hypercontractile esophagus, optimal management has yet to be determined, but treatment can include pharmacologic and endoscopic therapy [1–3]. Possible pharmacological approaches include proton pump inhibitors [4], calcium channel blockers [4], nitrates [4, 5], phosphodiesterase-5 inhibitors [5], anticholinergics [4, 6], and low-dose antidepressants [4]. Potential endoscopic approaches are botulinum toxin injection [4, 7], pneumatic dilation [4], and peroral endoscopic myotomy (POEM) [4, 8].

References

1. Monish R, Maheshawari A, Joshi R, et al. Vocal cord paralysis after cardiac surgery and interventions: a review of possible etiologies. J Cardiothorac Vasc Anesth. 2016;30(6):1661–7.
2. Clement M, Zhu W, Neshkova E, Bouin M. Jackhammer esophagus: from manometric diagnosis to clinical presentation. Can J Gastroenterol Hepatol. 2019;2019:1–7.
3. Tolone S, Savarino E, Docimo L. Radiofrequency catheter ablation for atrial fibrillation elicited "jackhammer esophagus": a new complication due to vagal nerve stimulation? J Neurogastroenterol Motil. 2015;21(4):612–5. https://doi.org/10.5056/jnm15034.
4. García-Lledó J, Clemente-Sánchez A, Merino-Rodríguez B, et al. Hypercontractile "jackhammer esophagus". Rev Esp Enferm Dig. 2015;107:234.
5. Schlottmann F, Patti M. Primary esophageal motility disorders: beyond achalasia. Int J Mol Sci. 2017;18(7):1399.
6. Jia Y, Arenas J, Hejazi RA, Elhanafi S, Saadi M, McCallum RW. Frequency of jackhammer esophagus as the extreme phenotypes of esophageal hypercontractility based on the new Chicago classification. J Clin Gastroenterol. 2016;50(8):615–8.
7. Marjoux S, Brochard C, Roman S, et al. Botulinum toxin injection for hypercontractile or spastic esophageal motility disorders: may high-resolution manometry help to select cases? Dis Esophagus. 2015;28(8):735–41.
8. Estremera-Arévalo F, Albéniz E, Rullán M, Areste I, Iglesias R, Vila J. Efficacy of peroral endoscopic myotomy compared with other invasive treatment options for the different esophageal motor disorders. Rev Esp Enferm Dig. 2017;109(8):578–86.

Unexpected Dysphagia and Heartburn After Neck Radiotherapy

Subhan Ahmad

1   Case Presentation

A 61-year-old female with a history of anal canal squamous cell carcinoma status post-chemoradiation, and progressive metastatic disease involving the cervical, supraclavicular, and mediastinal lymph nodes, pulmonary nodules, and tracheal mass requiring radiation therapy for neck adenopathy presented to the gastroenterology clinic for evaluation of dysphagia. She described food sticking at the level of the lower neck without associated weight loss, heartburn, odynophagia, or chest pain. A modified barium swallow study showed delayed passage of the barium cookie at the level of the vallecula. A barium esophagram showed a hiatal hernia and a large amount of induced gastroesophageal reflux. Esophagogastroduodenoscopy (EGD) showed a 2 cm sliding hiatal hernia, lax lower esophageal sphincter (LES), and circumferential erosive esophagitis in the proximal 3 cm of the esophagus consistent with radiation esophagitis (Fig. 1). The dysphagia was thought to be multifactorial and likely an oropharyngeal dysphagia, suspected gastroesphageal reflux disease (GERD), and radiation esophagitis in the proximal esophagus. She was instructed to take omeprazole 40 mg every morning and follow dysphagia precautions.

The patient returned to the clinic nearly two years later for evaluation of heartburn and ongoing dysphagia to solids and liquids. She endorsed symptoms of daily heartburn despite taking 40 mg of omeprazole twice daily and ranitidine 150 mg at bedtime. She described the dysphagia as a sensation of food getting stuck in her chest one to two times per week, usually when eating meat. She also reported coughing, choking, and occasional nausea with emesis, for which she occasionally

S. Ahmad (✉)
Division of Hospital Medicine, Case Western Reserve University School of Medicine, MetroHealth Medical Center, Cleveland, OH, USA
e-mail: sahmad1@metrohealth.org

R. Fass et al. (eds.), *Esophageal Disorders*,
https://doi.org/10.1007/978-3-031-56441-3_21

81

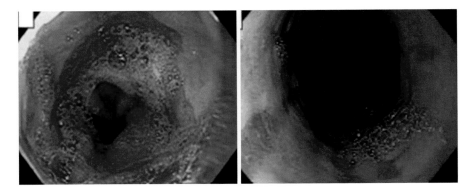

Fig. 1 Upper endoscopy showing normal z-line (left) but circumferential erosive esophagitis in the proximal 3 cm of the esophagus (right)

Fig. 2 Upper endoscopy showing whitish esophageal plaques and no luminal narrowing

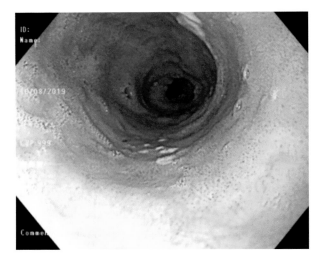

takes xyloxadryl oral solution but did not have odynophagia. Repeat EGD showed a 4 cm hiatal hernia, whitish esophageal plaques, and decreased esophageal peristaltic activity without any luminal narrowing (Fig. 2). Biopsies did not show evidence of eosinophilic esophagitis but did identify candida esophagitis, which was treated with fluconazole. As symptoms persisted, high-resolution esophageal manometry (HREM) was performed and showed normal median integrated relaxation pressure (IRP), borderline LES resting pressure, 50% weak swallows, and 50% failed swallows (Fig. 3). She was diagnosed with ineffective esophageal motility (IEM), and management of GERD was optimized with high-dose PPI and lifestyle changes as well as dysphagia precautions. She did well and regained her lost weight.

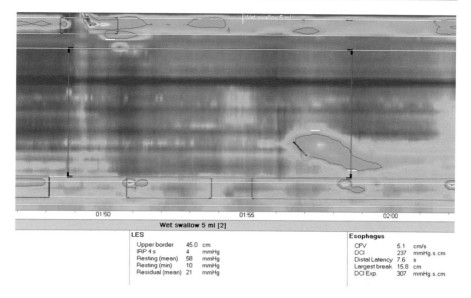

Wet swallow 5 ml [2]

LES			Esophagus		
Upper border	45.0	cm	CFV	5.1	cm/s
IRP 4 s	4	mmHg	DCI	237	mmHg.s.cm
Resting (mean)	58	mmHg	Distal Latency	7.6	s
Resting (min)	10	mmHg	Largest break	15.8	cm
Residual (mean)	21	mmHg	DCI Exp.	307	mmHg.s.cm

Fig. 3 High-resolution esophageal manometry showing a representative weak swallow. Tabular numbers pertain to this particular swallow

2 Discussion

Our patient had several potential etiologies of dysphagia. As suggested by the modi-fied barium swallow, oropharyngeal defects were present. Radiation esophagitis in the upper esophagus may have contributed as well. However, the clear symptom of esophageal dysphagia with the patient experiencing food sticking at the level of the chest suggested a problem in the more distal esophagus was the cause of the patient's symptoms. An investigation including upper endoscopy and HREM determined that the likely etiology of the patient's dysphagia was ineffective esophageal motility (IEM). IEM is an abnormality in peristaltic amplitude, contraction vigor, and/or peristaltic integrity with normal lower esophageal sphincter relaxation [1]. According to the Chicago Classification v4.0, at least 50% of swallows must be fol-lowed by failed contractions or more than 70% of swallows followed by ineffective contractions to meet diagnostic criteria [2].

IEM, the most common disorder identified on HREM, is found in 15–30% of patients undergoing the procedure, though the prevalence has lowered under the more stringent diagnostic criteria of Chicago Classification v4.0 [2]. Patients with IEM typically present with reflux-like symptoms or dysphagia. IEM is commonly discovered in patients with GERD, although which came first remains unknown [2–4]. Our patient had a large hiatal hernia and experienced heartburn that did not respond to standard dose PPI, making the link between GERD and IEM especially relevant to our patient. Had our patient experienced GERD symptoms that persisted despite high dose PPI, reflux testing to determine candidacy for more aggressive antireflux therapy, including antireflux surgery, would have been appropriate. Development of IEM after radiation therapy to the chest has not been previously described, and in our case it remains unknown whether radiation therapy triggered the development of IEM or the patient already had it.

The clinical significance of IEM is primarily that it may affect GERD treatment, specifically, patient's candidacy for endoscopic or surgical treatment of GERD. If our patient had been diagnosed with refractory GERD, the diagnosis of IEM would support pursuing a partial fundoplication, rather than a complete one, if antireflux surgery was to be pursued. However, IEM remains relevant on its own and can also be a cause of dysphagia even in the absence of GERD. Management of IEM is focused on optimizing treatment of GERD [5]. There is no effective treatment that can restore impaired smooth muscle contractility of the esophagus and thus improve symptoms [1–5].

References

1. Gyawali CP, Sifrim D, Carlson DA, et al. Ineffective esophageal motility: Concepts, future directions, and conclusions from the Stanford 2018 symposium. Neurogastroenterol Motil. 2019;31:e13584.
2. Yadlapati R, Kahrilas PJ, Fox MR, et al. Esophageal motility disorders on high-resolution manometry: Chicago classification version 4.0©. Neurogastroenterol Motil. 2021;33(1):e14058.
3. Scheerens C, Tack J, Rommel N. Buspirone, a new drug for the management of patients with ineffective esophageal motility? United Eur Gastroenterol J. 2015;3:261–5.
4. Kahrilas PJ, Bredenoord AJ, Fox M, et al. The chicago classification of esophageal motility disorders, v3.0. Neurogastroenterol Motil. 2015;27:160–74.
5. Triadafilopoulos G, Tandon A, Shetler KP, et al. Clinical and pH study characteristics in reflux patients with and without ineffective oesophageal motility (IEM). BMJ Open Gastroenterol. 2016;3:e000126.

Achalasia in a Poor Surgical Candidate

Subhan Ahmad

1 Case Presentation

An 82-year-old Caucasian male with known achalasia, diagnosed approximately 7 years ago, presented to the gastroenterology clinic with progressive worsening of dysphagia and regurgitation of solid and liquid foods several times a week. He endorsed a ten-pound weight loss in the past year and has had to sleep at an incline with bed wedges due to regurgitation of food at night. His past medical history is significant for colon cancer with a partial colectomy, coronary artery disease requiring percutaneous coronary intervention, peripheral vascular disease with prior femoral-popliteal bypass, and a transient ischemic attack. The patient was not treated at the time of diagnosis of achalasia due to his age and comorbidities and thus was advised to follow a soft diet. A timed barium esophagram showed a bird beak appearance of the distal esophagus, with less than 10% change in esophageal contrast volume between zero and five minutes as well as a large right epiphrenic esophageal diverticulum (Fig. 1).

An esophagogastroduodenoscopy (EGD) was completed which showed a large esophageal diverticulum, retained food in the esophagus and stomach, and resistance at the lower esophageal sphincter (LES) all consistent with the diagnosis of achalasia (Fig. 2). Due to his age and poor surgical candidacy, one hundred units of botulinum toxin were injected successfully, divided into four quadrants at the LES. Subsequent high-resolution esophageal manometry (HREM) showed 100% failed swallows and an integrated relaxation pressure (IRP) within normal range, but the test was non-diagnostic as the catheter appeared to enter the diverticulum rather than cross the LES (Fig. 3). The patient had a positive symptom response but

S. Ahmad (✉)
Division of Hospital Medicine, Case Western Reserve University School of Medicine, MetroHealth Medical Center, Cleveland, OH, USA
e-mail: sahmad1@metrohealth.org

© The Author(s), under exclusive license to Springer Nature Switzerland AG 2024
R. Fass et al. (eds.), *Esophageal Disorders*,
https://doi.org/10.1007/978-3-031-56441-3_22

Fig. 1 Barium esophagram showing a large right epiphrenic esophageal diverticulum

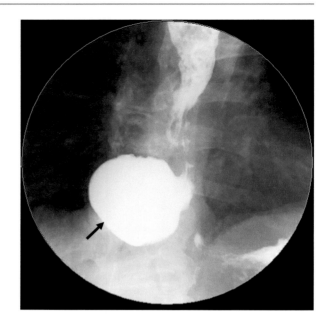

Fig. 2 EGD showing retained food in the esophagus

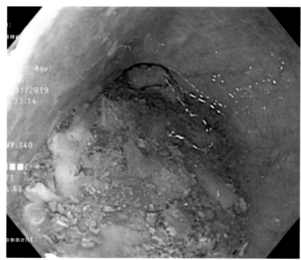

developed severe dysphagia again six months later. Repeat EGD with repeat Botulinum toxin injection into the LES was again performed. This time the patient had a near-complete response. Subsequent HREM showed a normalized IRP with scant peristaltic activity in the distal esophagus, consistent with successfully treated type 1 achalasia (Fig. 4).

Plans were made for further botulinum toxin injections as needed.

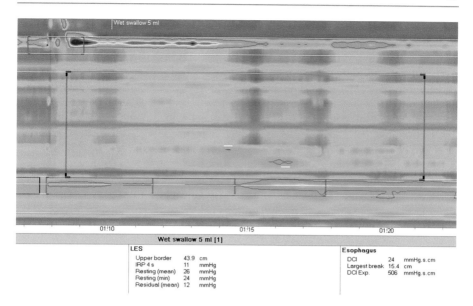

LES			Esophagus		
Upper border	43.9	cm	DCI	24	mmHg.s.cm
IRP 4 s	11	mmHg	Largest break	15.4	cm
Resting (mean)	26	mmHg	DCI Exp.	506	mmHg.s.cm
Resting (min)	24	mmHg			
Residual (mean)	12	mmHg			

Fig. 3 A representative swallow from high-resolution esophageal manometry showing no peristalsis but no definite pressure inversion, suggesting the catheter did not cross into the stomach. Tabular values pertain to this particular swallow

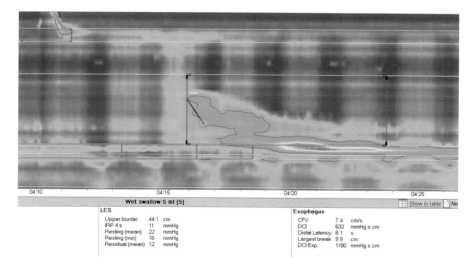

LES			Esophagus		
Upper border	44.1	cm	CFV	7.4	cm/s
IRP 4 s	11	mmHg	DCI	632	mmHg.s.cm
Resting (mean)	22	mmHg	Distal Latency	8.1	s
Resting (min)	16	mmHg	Largest break	9.9	cm
Residual (mean)	12	mmHg	DCI Exp.	1180	mmHg.s.cm

Fig. 4 A representative swallow from high-resolution esophageal manometry post-botulinum toxin injection therapy demonstrating a median IRP within the normal range, consistent with successfully treated type 1 achalasia, as well as development of peristaltic activity in the distal esophagus. Tabular values pertain to this particular swallow

2   Discussion

Although we have very definitive therapies for achalasia, such as pneumatic dilation, peroral endoscopic myotomy, and surgical myotomy, not all patients are candidates for these therapies. Our patient temporarily responded to a less invasive treatment option. Noninvasive management with oral medications or local botulinum toxin (BT) injection is considered in patients who are high-risk for a definitive interaction, like our patient [1, 2]. BT injection is the most effective, and commonly utilized, pharmacological therapy for achalasia. Injection into the LES inhibits the release of acetylcholine, causing smooth muscle relaxation and facilitating the passage of the food bolus into the gastric body. This is an effective short-term therapy; however, duration of effectiveness and need for repeat injections is variable but typically lasts between three and twelve months [2]. In some patients, the effect of BT injection may last longer. Our patient responded well in the short term, and BT injections can be repeated as needed.

References

1. Patel DA, Lappas BM, Vaezi MF. An overview of achalasia and its subtypes. Gastroenterol Hepatol (N Y). 2017;13(7):411–21.
2. Pasricha PJ, Rai R, Ravich WJ, Hendrix TR, Kalloo AN. Botulinum toxin for achalasia: long-term outcome and predictors of response. Gastroenterology. 1996;110(5):1410–5.

Two Disorders Wrapped into One

Subhan Ahmad

1   Case Presentation

A 58-year-old African American female presented for evaluation of dysphagia while undergoing presurgical evaluation for a laparoscopic sleeve gastrectomy. Her past medical history was significant for morbid obesity, well-controlled hypertension, hyperlipidemia, compensated chronic nonischemic systolic heart failure (ejection fraction 35%), obstructive sleep apnea, depression, osteoarthritis, and prediabetes. At the time of bariatric surgery evaluation, she complained of intermittent symptoms of esophageal dysphagia but had no symptoms of gastroesophageal reflux disease (GERD).

An upper endoscopy was performed and was unremarkable. She underwent high-resolution esophageal manometry (HREM), which showed an elevated median integrated relaxation pressure (IRP) in both supine and upright positions, abnormally high lower esophageal sphincter (LES) resting pressure, 60% normal swallows, and 40% hypercontractile swallows (Fig. 1). The patient was diagnosed with esophagogastric junction outflow obstruction (EGJOO) with hypercontractile esophagus. Given her symptoms were intermittent and relatively mild, no changes in her therapy were recommended, and she proceeded with bariatric surgery.

S. Ahmad (✉)
Division of Hospital Medicine, Case Western Reserve University School of Medicine, MetroHealth Medical Center, Cleveland, OH, USA
e-mail: sahmad1@metrohealth.org

© The Author(s), under exclusive license to Springer Nature Switzerland AG 2024
R. Fass et al. (eds.), *Esophageal Disorders*,
https://doi.org/10.1007/978-3-031-56441-3_23

89

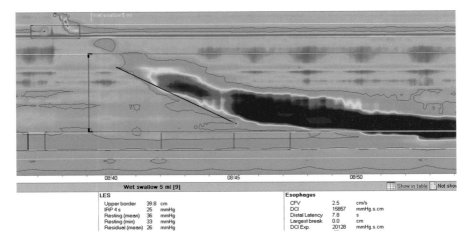

Fig. 1 A representative swallow from high-resolution esophageal manometry showing a hyper-contractile swallow with an elevated mean integrated relaxation pressure. Tabular numbers below pertain to this swallow

2   Discussion

Our patient has EGJOO with a hypercontractile esophagus. Based on the Chicago Classification v4.0, EGJOO criteria includes the presence of chest pain or dysphagia, and an elevated IRP that is persistent during both supine and upright positions with evidence of normal peristalsis. Supportive tests include a timed barium esophagram or an EndoFlip to evaluate the esophagogastric junction [1]. Our patient met the first two criteria but did not undergo any further testing to document the level of obstruction. However, an EGD was done and ruled out any mechanical obstruction that could explain her symptoms.

As seen in this patient, EGJOO is not always an exclusive diagnosis and has been reported concurrently with other motility disorders in up to 62% of patients [2]. It is now recognized that EGJOO can co-occur with other esophageal motility disorders, including hypercontractile esophagus, distal esophageal spasm, and ineffective esophageal motility [3]. Our patient had EGJOO with a hypercontractile esophagus. A possible explanation for this phenomenon is that the functional EGJOO can induce forceful contractions in the esophagus [3–5].

The diagnosis of EGJOO can sometimes be transient, and conservative management with observation and medical therapy for a period of six months is recommended in patients with recent onset or mild to moderate symptoms as seen in our patient [6].

References

1. Yadlapati R, Kahrilas PJ, Fox MR, et al. Esophageal motility disorders on high-resolution manometry: Chicago classification version 4.0©. Neurogastroenterol Motil. 2021;33(1):e14058. https://doi.org/10.1111/nmo.14058.
2. Richter JE, Clayton SB. Diagnosis and management of esophagogastric junction outflow obstruction. Am J Gastroenterol. 2019;114(4):544–7.
3. Schupack D, Katzka DA, Geno DM, Ravi K. The clinical significance of esophagogastric junction outflow obstruction and hypercontractile esophagus in high resolution esophageal manometry. Neurogastroenterol Motil. 2017;29(10):1–9.
4. Carlson DA, Kahrilas PJ, Lin Z, Hirano I, Gonsalves N, Listernick Z, Ritter K, Tye M, Ponds FA, Wong I, Pandolfino JE. Evaluation of esophageal motility utilizing the functional lumen imaging probe. Am J Gastroenterol. 2016;111(12):1726–35.
5. Yadlapati R, Kahrilas PJ. How updates in Chicago classification impact clinical practice. Foregut (Thousand Oaks). 2021;1(3):207–15.
6. Samo S, Qayed E. Esophagogastric junction outflow obstruction: where are we now in diagnosis and management? World J Gastroenterol. 2019;25(4):411–7. https://doi.org/10.3748/wjg.v25.i4.411.

Esophageal and Oropharyngeal Dysphagia

Subhan Ahmad

1 Case Presentation

A 66-year-old Caucasian female presented to the gastroenterology clinic for evaluation of chronic dysphagia and heartburn. She reported difficulty immediately after swallowing, with food getting stuck at the suprasternal notch. This mostly occurred after eating solids but sometimes happened with liquids as well. There was no associated chest pain or odynophagia. Her medical history was significant for hypertension, hyperlipidemia, migraines, and iron deficiency anemia. A barium esophagram showed high amplitude tertiary contractions in the distal esophagus suspicious for distal esophageal spasm, a cricopharyngeus bar, and a small sliding (type 1) hiatal hernia (Fig. 1). Her heartburn symptoms were well controlled on pantoprazole 40 mg daily.

High-resolution esophageal manometry (HREM) was obtained and showed normal median integrated relaxation pressure (IRP) (9.46 mmHg), normal lower esophageal sphincter (LES) resting pressure (32 mmHg), and 30% of swallows with simultaneous contractions, suspicious for distal esophageal spasm (DES) (Fig. 2). Although the distal latency was slightly above the cutoff to diagnose distal esophageal spasm by Chicago Classification v4.0, the appearance of a multiple simultaneous contractions in the distal esophagus paired with the classic corkscrew appearance on barium esophagram led to the decision to treat the patient medically for distal esophageal spasm. She was prescribed diltiazem 30 mg three to four times daily for a month and reported 40% improvement in swallowing. Her dose was increased to 60 mg four times per day, but this did not lead to any further improvement. She was referred to otolaryngology for her cricopharyngeal bar,

S. Ahmad (✉)
Division of Hospital Medicine, Case Western Reserve University School of Medicine, MetroHealth Medical Center, Cleveland, OH, USA
e-mail: sahmad1@metrohealth.org

© The Author(s), under exclusive license to Springer Nature Switzerland AG 2024
R. Fass et al. (eds.), *Esophageal Disorders*,
https://doi.org/10.1007/978-3-031-56441-3_24

Fig. 1 Barium esophagram showing high amplitude esophageal contractions with the classic corkscrew appearance of the distal esophagus, consistent with distal esophageal spasm

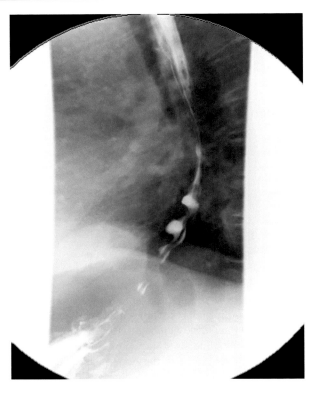

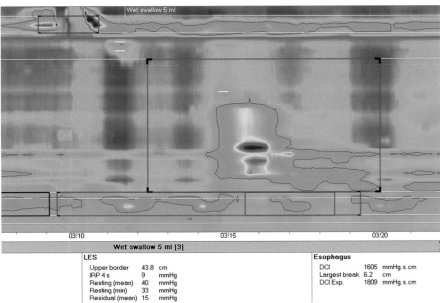

Fig. 2 Representative swallow from high-resolution esophageal manometry showing normal median integrated relaxation pressure and a simultaneous contraction of the distal esophagus. Tabular numbers are representative of this particular swallow

where a flexible esophagoscopy was performed and demonstrated a prominent cricopharyngeal bar that was dilated up to 57-French and injected with botulinum toxin. However, this too did not lead to improvement in her symptoms and she was referred back to gastroenterology for further management of her esophageal motility disorder. Repeat HREM continued to show simultaneous contractions of the distal esophagus but with normal distal latency. However, given ongoing suspicion for distal esophageal spasm that was persistent over a prolonged period and not responsive to medical therapy, the decision was made to treat the distal esophagus with botulinm toxin injection. After this, the patient experienced a resolution of her symptoms.

2   Discussion

The first step in evaluating patients presenting with nonacute dysphagia is to determine if the symptoms are due to oropharyngeal or esophageal dysphagia [1]. As described in this case, both etiologies could occur concomitantly. Without undergoing a comprehensive systematic evaluation, patients could be misdiagnosed and consequently not receive the appropriate treatment.

A thorough history can help distinguish between both etiologies with oropharyngeal dysphagia presenting as difficulty with initiating a swallow and is often accompanied by coughing, choking, and possible nasal regurgitation, while esophageal dysphagia presents with the sensation of food getting stuck a few seconds after initiating a swallow [1, 2]. Once the type of dysphagia is suspected based on history, further studies such as modified barium swallow, barium esophagram, esophagogastroduodenoscopy (EGD), and HREM can help with establishing the diagnosis.

This patient described food getting stuck at the level of the suprasternal notch immediately after swallowing. Her description has the characteristics of both oropharyngeal and esophageal dysphagia. Her HREM findings were consistent with the diagnosis of distal esophageal spasm (DES)—with a normal median IRP, normal LES resting pressure, and 30% simultaneous contractions. Her oropharyngeal dysphagia workup demonstrated a cricopharyngeal bar which was noted on a barium esophagram.

Our patient was initially treated pharmacologically for her DES with diltiazem 30 mg three to four times daily. She did experience considerable improvement with this treatment but had persistent symptoms. At that time, given the diagnosis of DES was not definite as well as the presence of oropharyngeal symptoms, treatment of the cricopharyngeal bar was attempted for both diagnostic and therapeutic purposes. Unfortunately, treatment of the cricopharyngeal bar with dilation and botulinm toxin injection did not lead to any symptomatic improvement. With more confidence that the patient's symptoms were due to her esophageal motility disorder, the decision was made to treat her suspected DES more aggressively with botulinm toxin injection into the distal esophagus. Ultimately, this led to resolution of her symptoms. Other therapies for DES include smooth muscle relaxants such as long-acting nitrates, anticholinergics, peppermint, neuromodulators, and invasive procedures such as botulinum toxin injections, peroral endoscopic myotomy, and long Heller myotomy [3].

References

1. Chilukuri P, Odufalu F, Hachem C. Dysphagia. Mo Med. 2018;115(3):206–10.
2. Gasiorowska A, Fass R. Current approach to dysphagia. Gastroenterol Hepatol. 2009;5:269.
3. Roman S, Kahrilas PJ. Management of spastic disorders of the esophagus. Gastroenterol Clin N Am. 2013 Mar;42(1):27–43.

Heartburn After Peroral Endoscopic Myotomy

Subhan Ahmad

1   Case Presentation

A 47-year-old male with a history of type 2 diabetes mellitus, hyperlipidemia, asthma, depression, and anxiety presented to the gastroenterology clinic for dysphagia. He described worsening dysphagia, heartburn, regurgitation of food two to three times per week, and nocturnal reflux symptoms despite appropriate proton pump inhibitor (PPI) therapy. A barium esophagram showed a small sliding-type hiatal hernia and mild gastroesophageal reflux. A pH impedance test was performed and showed adequate acid suppression with 69 weakly acidic reflux events (Fig. 1). The patient was referred for high-resolution esophageal manometry (HREM), which showed a high median integrated relaxation pressure (IRP), high lower esophageal sphincter (LES) resting pressure, 20% weak swallows, and 80% normal swallows (Fig. 2). He was diagnosed with esophagogastric junction outflow obstruction (EGJOO). CT scan was performed which showed no additional findings besides the known hiatal hernia. A gastric emptying study was also performed and showed 14% retention of gastric contents at four hours, consistent with borderline gastroparesis. The decision was made to proceed with peroral endoscopic myotomy (POEM) procedure as treatment of the EGJOO.

POEM was successfully completed, and his symptoms of dysphagia, heartburn, regurgitation of food, and nocturnal reflux symptoms improved. However, one year later the patient began to develop worsening reflux symptoms and regurgitation of food, particularly at nighttime, despite taking PPI twice daily and appropriate lifestyle modifications.

S. Ahmad (✉)
Division of Hospital Medicine, Case Western Reserve University School of Medicine, MetroHealth Medical Center, Cleveland, OH, USA
e-mail: sahmad1@metrohealth.org

1. PH (% time pH <4)

Upright   0
Supine   2.8
Total   1.2

2. Impedance

Total number of reflux events

	Acid	Weakly acid	Liquid	Mixed	Total
Upright	1	63	14	53	67
Supine	4	6	10	0	10
Total	5	69	24	53	77

3) Indices

SI   0

SAP   0

Conclusions:

1. Normal pH test
2. Abnormal impedance (weakly acidic reflux) but inconclusive reflux burden
3. Negative symptom indexes

Fig. 1 Impedance + PH test results showing normal esophageal acid exposure, a borderline number of reflux events with negative symptom association

HREM was repeated and now showed normal median IRP, normal LES basal pressure, 10% failed swallows, and 90% weak swallows consistent with ineffective esophageal motility (Fig. 3). An EGD was also repeated and showed LA grade C erosive esophagitis (Fig. 4). He was continued on PPI twice daily in addition to sucralfate and an evening dose of ranitidine. Despite the increased acid suppression, the patient had persistent reflux symptoms and ultimately decided to undergo laparoscopic hiatal hernia repair with Toupet fundoplication. He did well after surgery with resolution of his symptoms.

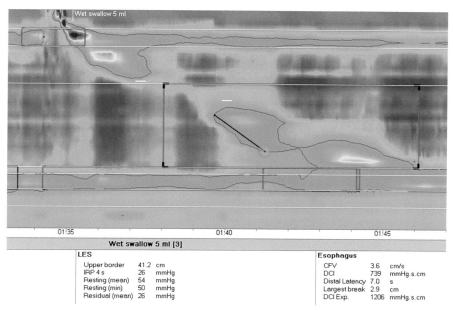

Fig. 2 A representative swallow from high-resolution esophageal manometry (pre-treatment) showing a high median integrated relaxation pressure and normal peristalsis. Tabular numbers below pertain to this swallow

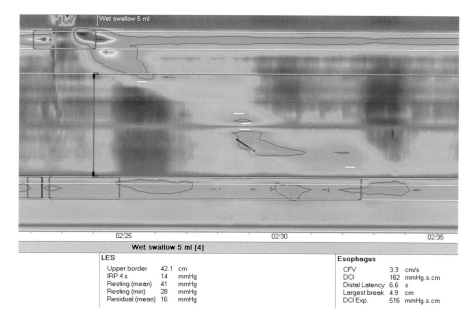

Fig. 3 A representative swallow from high-resolution esophageal manometry after POEM showing a normalized median integrated relaxation pressure and a weak swallow, consistent with ineffective esophageal motility. Tabular numbers below pertain to this swallow

Fig. 4 EGD showing LA
grade C erosive esophagitis

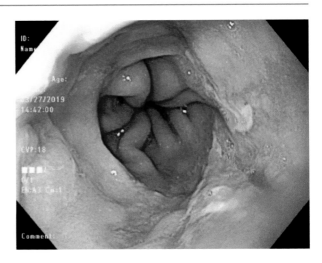

2   Discussion

POEM is an increasingly popular treatment of symptomatic, manometry-proven, esophageal motility disorders [1, 2]. It is the endoscopic, less invasive, equivalent of surgical myotomy that involves tunneling into the submucosal layer of the esophagus and proximal stomach through which esophageal and gastric myotomy are performed using a flexible endoscope [1]. In addition to its widely accepted use in achalasia, POEM has also been successfully used as the primary treatment of other esophageal motility disorders, such as EGJOO, diffuse esophageal spasm, and hypercontractile esophagus [2, 3]. In our case, this patient underwent POEM for EGJOO with successful resolution of his dysphagia.

Early complications after POEM include mucosal injury (4.8%), subcutaneous emphysema (7.5%), and pneumoperitoneum (6.8%) [2–5]. The most common late complication seen post-POEM is gastroesophageal reflux disease (GERD) (16–21%), which typically occurs two to three months postoperatively [2, 3]. Most patients can be managed effectively with PPIs [6]. Unfortunately, our patient experienced refractory GERD as a complication of his POEM procedure. The borderline gastroparesis and IEM may have contributed to his GERD being especially difficult to control. Thankfully, antireflux surgery was successful in resolving these symptoms without causing a recurrence of dysphagia.

References

1. Khashab MA, Pasricha PJ. Conquering the third space: challenges and opportunities for diagnostic and therapeutic endoscopy. Gastrointest Endosc. 2013;77:146.
2. Kim JY, Min YW. Peroral endoscopic Myotomy for esophageal motility disorders. Clin Endosc. 2020;53(6):638–45. https://doi.org/10.5946/ce.2020.223.

3. Inoue H, Minami H, Kobayashi Y, et al. Peroral endoscopic myotomy (POEM) for esophageal achalasia. Endoscopy. 2010;42:265–71.
4. Hernández-Mondragón OV, Solórzano-Pineda OM, González-Martínez MA, Blancas-Valencia JM, Caballero-Luengas C. Peroral endoscopic myotomy for the treatment of achalasia and other esophageal motor disorders: short-term and medium-term results at a Mexican tertiary care center. Rev Gastroenterol Mex. 2019;84:1–10.
5. Cho YK, Kim SH. Current status of peroral endoscopic myotomy. Clin Endosc. 2018;51:13–8.
6. Talukdar R, Inoue H, Nageshwar RD. Efficacy of peroral endoscopic myotomy (POEM) in the treatment of achalasia: a systematic review and meta-analysis. Surg Endosc. 2015;29:3030–46.

Dysphagia and Connective Tissue Disease

Subhan Ahmad

1 Case Presentation

A 60-year-old African American female presented to the gastroenterology clinic for a follow-up regarding dysphagia, diarrhea, and abdominal pain. Her medical history was significant for limited scleroderma (treated with mycophenolate mofetil), hypertension, coronary artery disease, chronic obstructive pulmonary disease, nicotine and cannabis use disorder, and history of cholecystectomy. Dysphagia, particularly when initiating a swallow, was reported to occur up to five times per month, usually with solid foods, liquids, pills, and saliva. Diarrhea was chronic, intermittent in nature with some improvement with loperamide. The patient reported periumbilical pain as well as lower abdominal pain lasting about one week every month, not associated with diarrhea, and improved with dicyclomine. She had no weight loss, nausea, vomiting, gastrointestinal bleeding, or recent changes in medications.

An esophagogastroduodenoscopy (EGD) and colonoscopy were normal except for five polyps in the transverse and descending colon which were removed. Biopsies of the esophagus and colon were unremarkable.

Symptoms persisted over several months and further testing was performed. Barium esophagram showed a small, two cm, self-reducing, sliding (type I) hiatal hernia as well as large volume, spontaneous reflux to the level of the thoracic inlet. High-resolution esophageal manometry (HREM) showed normal median integrated relaxation pressure (IRP), normal lower esophageal sphincter (LES) resting pressure, 10% failed swallows, 70% weak swallows, and a hiatal hernia (Fig. 1). She was diagnosed with ineffective esophageal motility (IEM) and was educated about

S. Ahmad (✉)
Division of Hospital Medicine, Case Western Reserve University School of Medicine, MetroHealth Medical Center, Cleveland, OH, USA
e-mail: sahmad1@metrohealth.org

© The Author(s), under exclusive license to Springer Nature Switzerland AG 2024
R. Fass et al. (eds.), *Esophageal Disorders*,
https://doi.org/10.1007/978-3-031-56441-3_26

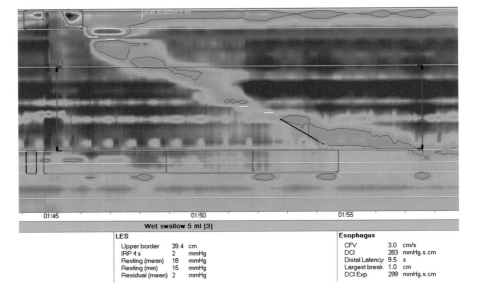

LES			Esophagus		
Upper border	39.4	cm	CFV	3.0	cm/s
IRP 4 s	2	mmHg	DCI	283	mmHg.s.cm
Resting (mean)	18	mmHg	Distal Latency	9.5	s
Resting (min)	15	mmHg	Largest break	1.0	cm
Residual (mean)	2	mmHg	DCI Exp.	299	mmHg.s.cm

Fig. 1 Representative swallow from high-resolution esophageal manometry showing a weak swallow with normal median integrated relaxation pressure. Tabular values below pertain to this swallow

dysphagia precautions and started on famotidine 40 mg daily. In follow-up one year later, her symptoms were well-controlled.

2   Discussion

Limited cutaneous systemic sclerosis is a subtype of systemic sclerosis (SSc), a multisystem autoimmune connective tissue disorder. This form of systemic sclerosis is often associated with CREST (calcinosis cutis, raynaud phenomenon, esophageal dysmotility, sclerodactyly, and telangiectasia) syndrome. Common forms of esophageal dysmotility in scleroderma are absent contractility and IEM. Diagnostic evaluation begins with upper endoscopy and can include reflux testing and barium esophagram. HREM is the preferred tool for diagnosis of associated esophageal motility disorders. Our patient was diagnosed with IEM, which on manometry is characterized by ineffective swallows, often with poor bolus transit in the distal esophagus [1, 2].

Treatment of IEM in patients with SSc is supportive. Patients are advised to chew well, avoid large bites, and drink water following swallows of solid food. Acid suppression is often utilized given the common presence of comorbid gastroesophageal reflux disease (GERD). Our patient's symptoms improved with these dietary recommendations and acid suppression with an H2 receptor antagonist. In many patients, more aggressive acid suppression with proton pump inhibitors (PPIs) is required

[3]. Other potential treatments include buspirone, a 5-hydroxytryptamine 1A receptor agonist, which has shown promising beneficial effects in patients with IEM and heartburn or regurgitation, though no improvement was seen with dysphagia and chest pain [4]. Although there is limited evidence to support their use, some practitioners will prescribe a prokinetic agent in patients with absent contractility or ineffective esophageal motility whose symptoms persist despite high-dose PPI [5]. Prevention of scleroderma progression with immunomodulators would theoretically slow down progression of gastrointestinal manifestations; however, more studies are needed to confirm this. The use of antireflux surgery for refractory cases is controversial, but some data suggests that partial fundoplication can be effective at reducing reflux without increasing postoperative dysphagia [6].

References

1. Ebert EC. Esophageal disease in scleroderma. J Clin Gastroenterol. 2006;40:769–75.
2. Ntoumazios SK, Voulgari PV, Potsis K, Koutis E, Tsifetaki N, Assimakopoulos DA. Esophageal involvement in scleroderma: gastroesophageal reflux, the common problem. Semin Arthritis Rheum. 2006;36:173–81.
3. Denaxas K, Ladas SD, Karamanolis GP. Evaluation and management of esophageal manifestations in systemic sclerosis. Ann Gastroenterol. 2018;31(2):165–70. https://doi.org/10.20524/aog.2018.0228.
4. Karamanolis GP, Panopoulos S, Denaxas K, et al. The 5-HT1A receptor agonist buspirone improves esophageal motor function and symptoms in systemic sclerosis:a 4-week, open-label trial. Arthritis Res Ther. 2016;18:195.
5. Voulgaris TA, Karamanolis GP. Esophageal manifestation in patients with scleroderma. World J Clin Cases. 2021;9(20):5408–19.
6. Seo KW, Park MI, Yoon KY, Park SJ, Kim SE. Laparoscopic partial fundoplication in case of gastroesophageal reflux disease patient with absent esophageal motility. J Gastric Cancer. 2015;15(2):127–31.

GERD That Would Not Get Better

Sara Kamionkowski

1   Case Presentation

A 55-year-old female initially presented to the gastroenterology clinic with complaints of persistent heartburn. She had a complicated medical history including chronic lymphocytic leukemia, diffuse large B-cell lymphoma, graft versus host disease after allogeneic stem cell transplant, and recurrent venous thromboembolisms. She had previously been treated with chemotherapy and radiation almost 20 years prior to her presentation. Other than heartburn, her symptoms also included regurgitation of food that was worse at nighttime. She denied dysphagia and reported that her symptoms persisted for about 18 months. She had tried taking ranitidine, omeprazole twice daily, sucralfate, esomeprazole, and calcium carbonate, but none had been effective in relieving her symptoms. An upper endoscopy revealed LA grade C erosive esophagitis (Fig. 1). She underwent pH impedance testing on omeprazole 40 mg twice daily, which demonstrated an elevated acid exposure time (AET) of 10.7% in the upright position, and abnormally high weakly acidic reflux with a total of 69 events over 24 h. Her PPI was switched to dexlansoprazole 60 mg daily and baclofen 10 mg at bedtime was added. Despite this, her symptoms persisted. She underwent high-resolution esophageal manometry (HREM), which showed 100% failed swallows with a normal integrated relaxation pressure (IRP) and normal lower esophageal sphincter (LES) resting pressure (Fig. 2). She was diagnosed with absent contractility. Lifestyle changes including sleeping upright and avoiding food or liquids before bedtime were reinforced, and her dose of baclofen was increased to 10 mg twice daily. Sucralfate and buspirone 5 mg daily

S. Kamionkowski (✉)
Department of Gastroenterology and Hepatology, Case Western Reserve University School of Medicine, MetroHealth Medical Center, Cleveland, OH, USA
e-mail: skamionkowski@metrohealth.org

© The Author(s), under exclusive license to Springer Nature   107
Switzerland AG 2024
R. Fass et al. (eds.), *Esophageal Disorders*,
https://doi.org/10.1007/978-3-031-56441-3_27

Fig. 1 EGD showing LA
grade C erosive esophagitis

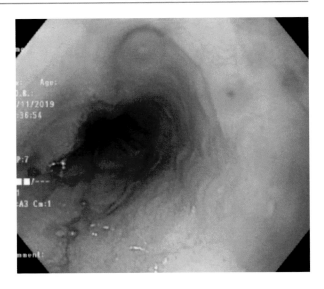

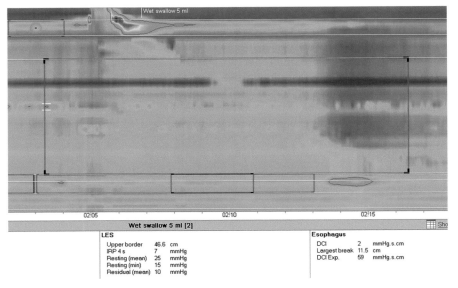

LES			Esophagus		
Upper border	46.6	cm	DCI	2	mmHg.s.cm
IRP 4 s	7	mmHg	Largest break	11.5	cm
Resting (mean)	25	mmHg	DCI Exp.	59	mmHg.s.cm
Resting (min)	15	mmHg			
Residual (mean)	10	mmHg			

Fig. 2 Representative swallow from high-resolution esophageal manometry showing a failed
swallow with a low lower esophageal sphincter pressure. Tabular values below represent this
swallow only

were also added to her treatment regimen. With these changes she did experience
some improvement in her symptoms.

2 Discussion

Absent contractility is a disorder of esophageal hypomotility characterized by the complete absence of any peristaltic activity in the esophagus following a swallow, in the absence of an esophagogastric junction outlet disorder [1, 2]. Absent contractility may be associated with rheumatologic and connective tissue disorders [3], which were not detected in our patient. It is unclear whether her history of radiation or chemotherapy could have contributed to her diagnosis; however, there are no studies that have reported such an association.

Patients with absent contractility often have GERD that is difficult to control, as the absence of primary and secondary peristalsis can lead to prolonged reflux events [4]. Treatment recommendations focus on aggressive GERD management and include acid suppression using high dose PPIs or a combination of high dose PPI and H2 blocker, as well as lifestyle modifications such as sleeping upright, on the left side, and avoiding oral intake at least 3 h prior to bedtime. Other agents used adjunctively to PPIs include buspirone and baclofen, which are thought to improve esophageal motor function or decrease the number of transient LES relaxations, respectively [5]. In our case, maximizing medical management resulted in some improvement in her symptoms.

References

1. Yadlapati R, Kahrilas PJ, Fox MR, Bredenoord AJ, Gyawali CP, Roman S, Babaei A, Mittal RK, Rommel N, Savarino E, et al. Esophageal motility disorders on high-resolution manometry: Chicago classification version 4.0©. Neurogastroenterol Motil. 2021;33:e14058.
2. Kahrilas PJ, Bredenoord AJ, Fox M, et al. The Chicago classification of esophageal motility disorders, v3.0. Neurogastroenterol Motil. 2015;27(2):160–74. https://doi.org/10.1111/nmo.12477.
3. Laique S, Singh T, Dornblaser D, Gadre A, Rangan V, Fass R, Kirby D, Chatterjee S, Gabbard S. Clinical characteristics and associated systemic diseases in patients with esophageal "absent contractility"—a clinical algorithm. J Clin Gastroenterol. 2019;53:184–90.
4. Cohen DL, Dickman R, Bermont A, Richter V, Shirin H, Mari A. The natural history of esophageal "absent contractility" and its relationship with rheumatologic diseases: a multi-center case–control study. J Clin Med. 2022;11(13):3922. https://doi.org/10.3390/jcm11133922.
5. Blonski W, Vela MF, Freeman J, Sharma N, Castell DO. The effect of oral buspirone, pyridostigmine, and bethanechol on esophageal function evaluated with combined multichannel esophageal impedance-manometry in healthy volunteers. J Clin Gastroenterol. 2009;43(3):253–60. https://doi.org/10.1097/MCG.0b013e318167b89d.

Heartburn Without Reflux

Yeseong Kim

1   Case Description

A 32-year-old woman with morbid obesity, generalized anxiety disorder, obsessive-compulsive disorder, obstructive sleep apnea, and irritable bowel syndrome (IBS) presented to the esophageal and swallowing center for reflux symptoms. Specifically, she was experiencing epigastric pain, heartburn, throat burning, and a lot of phlegm that required frequent throat clearing. She also noted unintentional weight loss of 25 pounds over 3 months but denied anorexia, dysphagia, or odynophagia. She was taking omeprazole 40 mg twice daily and ranitidine 300 mg at bedtime but had persistent symptoms. A nasolaryngoscopy demonstrated laryngeal changes that are suspected to be due to laryngopharyngeal reflux. The patient underwent EGD with wireless pH capsule placement after discontinuing omeprazole. Other than a 3 cm hiatal hernia, there were no endoscopic abnormalities (Fig. 1). Results of the wireless pH test showed an acid exposure time (AET) within the physiologic range and no correlation between reflux events and symptoms (Fig. 2). The patient was diagnosed with functional heartburn. She resumed her PPI and started on low-dose nortriptyline with improvement in her symptoms.

Y. Kim (✉)
Division of Gastroenterology and Hepatology, Lewis Katz School of Medicine at Temple University, Temple University Hospital, Philadelphia, PA, USA

© The Author(s), under exclusive license to Springer Nature Switzerland AG 2024
R. Fass et al. (eds.), *Esophageal Disorders*,
https://doi.org/10.1007/978-3-031-56441-3_28

Fig. 1 Upper endoscopy of the patient showing normal gastroesophageal junction

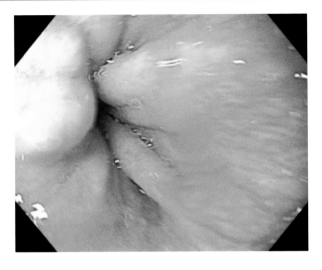

Days	Fraction time pH < 4 (%)		
	Upright	Supine	Total
Day #1	3.4	0.8	2.3
Day #2	4.5	0	3.4
Combined	4.0	0.5	2.8

	Heartburn	Chest Pain	Regurgitation
SI	0	0	5.6
SAP	0	0	0

Fig. 2 Wireless pH tests showing a normal esophageal acid exposure time along with no correlation between reflux events and symptoms

2 Discussion

This patient presented with refractory reflux-like symptoms, as she experienced heartburn that did not improve despite high-dose proton pump inhibitor (PPI). In patients such as this with reflux symptoms who do not have history of proven GERD, they should first undergo an upper endoscopy and, if negative, reflux testing off PPI treatment to rule out objective GERD. While catheter-based pH and pH impedance testing are reasonable options, wireless pH capsule testing is the preferred modality due to a higher sensitivity at detecting objective GERD [1]. This test should be performed after the patient has discontinued PPI use for 7 days. As with our patient, if this testing reveals a physiologic amount of acid reflux while off of acid-suppressing medications, GERD is ruled out, and a functional esophageal disorder can be suspected. Functional heartburn (FH) is differentiated from reflux hypersensitivity (RH) in that patients with RH have a positive association between their symptoms and reflux events, in the absence of pathologic acid reflux [2]. Esophageal manometry should also be performed prior to confirming the diagnosis to rule out an esophageal motility disorder.

FH is characterized by the experience of heartburn in the absence of objective evidence of GERD or any other esophageal disorder that explains the reflux symptoms [1, 2]. FH, like many other disorders of gut-brain interactions (DGBIs), has a young female predominance [3, 4]. FH constitutes approximately 21% of all untreated patients presenting with heartburn [5, 6]. Patients with FH often present with similar complaints as do patients with GERD and often have other disorders of gut-brain interactions (DGBIs), such as functional dysphagia, functional dyspepsia, and irritable bowel syndrome (IBS) [6]. Pathophysiological studies involving esophageal balloon distension and electrical stimulation of the esophagus have shown that FH is primarily driven by esophageal hypersensitivity [7, 8]. Neuromodulators such as tricyclic antidepressants and selective serotonin reuptake inhibitors are commonly used as pharmacologic therapy, while non-pharmacologic options include hypnotherapy, acupuncture, and psychological intervention such as mindfulness and cognitive behavioral therapy [9]. Our patient responded well to the addition of a low-dose TCA. However, an attempt to discontinue the PPI should have been considered.

References

1. Yamasaki T, O'Neil J, Fass R. Update on functional heartburn. Gastroenterol Hepatol. 2017;13(12):725.
2. Blaga TS, Dumitrascu D, Galmiche J-P, des Varannes SB. Functional heartburn: clinical characteristics and outcome. Eur J Gastroenterol Hepatol. 2013;25(3):282–90.
3. Savarino E, Pohl D, Zentilin P, et al. Functional heartburn has more in common with functional dyspepsia than with non-erosive reflux disease. Gut. 2009;58(9):1185–91.
4. De Bortoli N, Frazzoni L, Savarino EV, et al. Functional heartburn overlaps with irritable bowel syndrome more often than GERD. Am J Gastroenterol. 2016;111(12):1711–7.
5. Kondo T, Miwa H. The role of esophageal hypersensitivity in functional heartburn. J Clin Gastroenterol. 2017;51(7):571–8.
6. Fass R. Functional heartburn: what it is and how to treat it. Gastrointest Endosc Clin N Am. 2009;19(1):23–33.
7. Fass R, Tougas G. Functional heartburn: the stimulus, the pain, and the brain. Gut. 2002;51(6):885–92.
8. Yang M, Li Z-s, Chen D-f, et al. Quantitative assessment and characterization of visceral hyperalgesia evoked by esophageal balloon distention and acid perfusion in patients with functional heartburn, nonerosive reflux disease, and erosive esophagitis. Clin J Pain. 2010;26(4):326–31.
9. Riehl ME, Pandolfino JE, Palsson OS, Keefer L. Feasibility and acceptability of esophageal-directed hypnotherapy for functional heartburn. Dis Esophagus. 2016;29(5):490–6.

Resolution of Dysphagia Post-peroral Endoscopic Myotomy

Sara Ghoneim

1 Case Presentation

A 48-year-old African American female with morbid obesity and type 2 diabetes mellitus was referred to the gastroenterology clinic because of progressive dysphagia. She was otherwise well until 2 years ago when she developed dysphagia to solids, liquids, and pills occurring at least three to four times a week. Her dysphagia was associated with coughing and choking events prompting her to seek medical care. She underwent an upper endoscopy which revealed a tortuous esophagus (Fig. 1). Esophageal biopsies were negative for eosinophilic esophagitis. She then underwent high-resolution esophageal manometry (HREM), which showed elevated lower esophageal sphincter (LES) resting pressure, high median integrated relaxation pressure (IRP), no peristalsis, and spastic contractions occurring in 30% of swallows (Fig. 2). These findings were suggestive of type 3 achalasia. A timed barium esophagram demonstrated mild esophageal dilation with a bird beak appearance at the esophagogastric junction (EGJ). Moderate contrast retention was seen at the level of the aortic arch, but minimal contrast residual was left in the esophagus at 5 min. Passage of a 1.3 cm barium tablet was impeded at the level of the EGJ. The patient elected to undergo POEM. EndoFLIP was used during the procedure to compare area and distensibility before (Fig. 3) and after (Table 1) the esophageal myotomy, and a large improvement was noticed. Endoscopic examination at the end of the procedure revealed widely patent GEJ, and the patient reported complete resolution of her symptoms.

S. Ghoneim (✉)
Department of Gastroenterology and Hepatology, University of Nebraska College of Medicine, University of Nebraska Medical Center, Omaha, NE, USA

© The Author(s), under exclusive license to Springer Nature Switzerland AG 2024
R. Fass et al. (eds.), *Esophageal Disorders*,
https://doi.org/10.1007/978-3-031-56441-3_29

Fig. 1 Upper endoscopy
showing a tortuous
esophagus

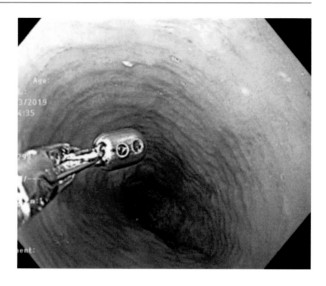

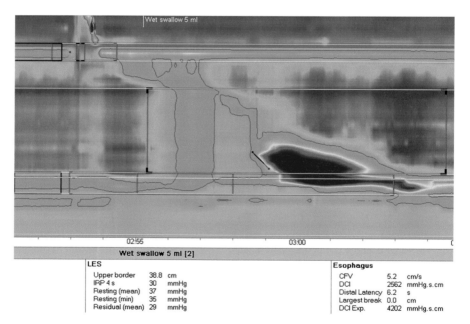

LES			Esophagus		
Upper border	38.8	cm	CFV	5.2	cm/s
IRP 4 s	30	mmHg	DCI	2562	mmHg.s.cm
Resting (mean)	37	mmHg	Distal Latency	6.2	s
Resting (min)	35	mmHg	Largest break	0.0	cm
Residual (mean)	29	mmHg	DCI Exp.	4202	mmHg.s.cm

Fig. 2 Representative swallow from high-resolution esophageal manometry showing a high median integrated relaxation pressure, no organized peristalsis, and spastic simultaneous contraction of the esophagus. Tabular numbers below are representative of this particular swallow

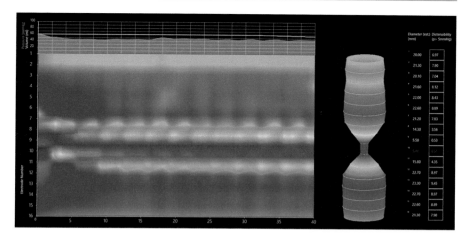

Fig. 3 Pre-treatment EndoFLIP evaluation showing low distensibility index and diameter at a volume of 60mL

Table 1 Posttreatment EndoFLIP evaluation

Balloon size (cc)	Diameter (mm)	Distensibility index (mm²/mmHg)
40	8	2.5
50	12.5	4.5
Repetitive antegrade contractions		No
Contraction pattern		Minimal contractions
Balloon pressure >15		Yes

2   Discussion

Here we describe a case of patient presenting with dysphagia to solids and liquids who was eventually diagnosed with type III achalasia: an esophageal motility disorder characterized by incomplete LES relaxation in the setting of absent esophageal peristalsis [1]. According to Chicago Classification v4.0, a conclusive diagnosis of type 3 achalasia, which is the diagnosis of our patient, is defined by an abnormal IRP and evidence of spasm (20% or more swallows with premature contraction) with no evidence of peristalsis [2]. Of the achalasia subtypes, type 3 achalasia is typically the least likely to respond to surgical or endoscopic therapy, though POEM is the preferred treatment modality due to the ability to extend the myotomy above the LES to the distal esophagus which is the site of spastic contractions [4]. Our patient responded well to POEM.

The endoluminal functional lumen imaging probe (EndoFLIP®), a device that can measure cross-sectional area, intraluminal pressure, and intraluminal distensibility of the esophagus [3], has several important uses in patients with achalasia or suspected achalasia. First, it serves as another supportive diagnostic test for patients in whom the diagnosis is unclear or who do not tolerate HREM. Furthermore, as happened in our case, it can also be used perioperatively to predict the success of a POEM procedure, by comparing the area and distensibility of the LES before and after the procedure.

References

1. Pandolfino JE, Gawron AJ. Achalasia: a systematic review. JAMA. 2015;313(18):1841–52.
2. Yadlapati R, Kahrilas PJ, Fox MR, et al. Esophageal motility disorders on high-resolution manometry: Chicago classification version 4.0©. Neurogastroenterol Motil. 2021;33(1):e14058.
3. Kim GH. Is EndoFLIP useful for predicting clinical outcomes after peroral endoscopic myotomy in patients with achalasia? Gut Liver. 2019;13(1):3–4.
4. Kumbhari V, Tieu AH, Onimaru M, et al. Peroral endoscopic myotomy (POEM) vs laparoscopic Heller myotomy (LHM) for the treatment of type III achalasia in 75 patients: a multicenter comparative study. Endosc Int Open. 2015;3(3):E195–201.

Recurrent Dysphagia After Nissen Fundoplication

Sara Kamionkowski

1   Case Presentation

A 69-year-old male with remote history of Nissen fundoplication, diabetes, chronic kidney disease, prostate cancer status post-prostatectomy with salvage radiation, hypertension, and hyperlipidemia presented to the gastroenterology clinic for a barium esophagram that incidentally showed a stricture at the esophagogastric junction (EGJ) with pooling of contrast within the esophagus. He subsequently underwent esophagogastroduodenoscopy (EGD) that revealed an akinetic, dilated esophagus with LA grade C erosive esophagitis (Fig. 1). Empirical balloon dilation to 18 mm was performed at the EGJ, but this did not lead to improvement in symptoms. He then underwent high-resolution esophageal manometry (HREM), which demonstrated an elevated median integrated relaxation pressure (IRP) (49 mmHg), mean lower esophageal sphincter (LES) resting pressure (54 mmHg), and 100% failed swallows. His findings were consistent with a diagnosis of achalasia, type 1 (Fig. 2). He had a repeat EGD with successful fluoroscopic guided 30 mm pneumatic balloon dilation. This initially led to symptom relief for 6 months, but afterward his symptoms returned and gradually worsened over several years until he began experiencing regurgitation and vomiting of undigested food. Subsequent repeat timed barium esophagogram (TBE) showed dilated esophagus with narrowing at the EGJ and moderate amount of residual contrast that remained unchanged after 5 min. Repeat EGD with EndoFLIP showed normal appearing mucosa but dilated esophagus without contractions and a tight LES. The patient was offered peroral endoscopic myotomy (POEM); however, he declined the procedure and

S. Kamionkowski (✉)
Department of Gastroenterology and Hepatology, Case Western Reserve University School of Medicine, MetroHealth Medical Center, Cleveland, OH, USA
e-mail: skamionkowski@metrohealth.org

© The Author(s), under exclusive license to Springer Nature Switzerland AG 2024
R. Fass et al. (eds.), *Esophageal Disorders*,
https://doi.org/10.1007/978-3-031-56441-3_30

119

Fig. 1 Dilated distal
esophagus with esophagitis

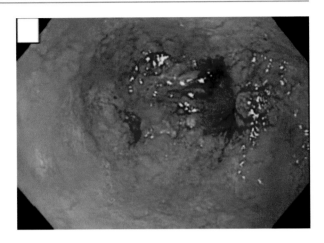

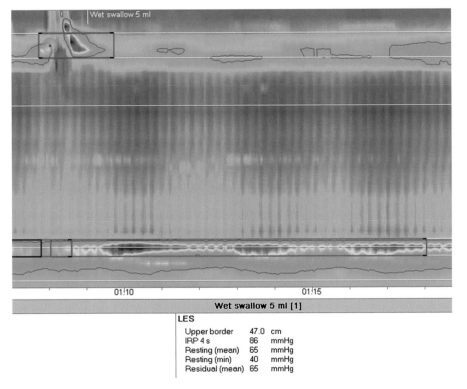

LES		
Upper border	47.0	cm
IRP 4 s	86	mmHg
Resting (mean)	65	mmHg
Resting (min)	40	mmHg
Residual (mean)	65	mmHg

Fig. 2 Representative swallow from the high-resolution esophageal manometry showing a failed swallow and impaired relaxation of the lower esophageal sphincter. Tabular numbers below pertain to this swallow

reported improvement in his symptoms with lifestyle changes including small, frequent meals and by elevating the head of the bed at night.

2 Discussion

Type 1 (classic) achalasia is defined manometrically by an abnormally high median IRP and no esophageal contractility (100% failed peristalsis) [1]. Pharmacologic treatment of achalasia has limited efficacy [2], and invasive therapy is the mainstay of treatment. The three first-line treatment options are pneumatic dilation, peroral endoscopic myotomy (POEM), and laparoscopic Heller myotomy with partial fundoplication. These three options are thought to have similar efficacy with good durability of at least 5–10 years [2]. In our case the patient underwent pneumatic dilation to 30 mm but then developed a gradual return of symptoms over 6 months. This may have occurred due to incomplete dilation. Pneumatic dilation can be offered as "graded dilation," in which several dilations at increasing balloon diameters, to a maximum of 40 mm, are scheduled, in order to achieve long-lasting response. An alternative approach is "as needed" dilations, in which dilations can be performed repeatedly at a diameter of 30 mm, 35 mm, or 40 mm, as the patient redevelops symptoms [3]. Alternatively, POEM or Heller myotomy can be performed if symptoms recur after pneumatic dilation. Currently there is insufficient data to recommend any of these approaches over the others, and any approach is reasonable [3]. Unfortunately, our patient declined referral for an effective long-term therapy of achalasia and given the progressive nature of the disease is at risk of experiencing a worsening of his symptoms over time that may no longer respond to the lifestyle measures he has adopted.

References

1. Riccio F, Costantini M, Salvador R. Esophageal achalasia: diagnostic evaluation. World J Surg. 2022;46:1516–21.
2. Schlottmann F, Herbella F, et al. Modern management of esophageal achalasia: from pathophysiology to treatment. Curr Probl Surg. 2018;55:10–37.
3. Khashab MA, Vela MF, Thosani N, et al. ASGE guideline on the management of achalasia. Gastrointest Endosc. 2020;91(2):213–227.e6.

Dysphagia and Chest Pain in a Patient with Emphysema

Sara Kamionkowski

1 Case Presentation

A 62-year-old female with a past medical history of chronic obstructive pulmonary disease (COPD) and tobacco use disorder presented initially to her primary care doctor with 4 years of midepigastric pain and non-cardiac chest pain when swallowing either solids or liquids. She was started on twice daily esomeprazole 40 mg but the symptoms persisted. She was also referred for an esophagogastroduodenoscopy (EGD), which was normal, including esophageal biopsies. She then underwent a barium esophagram, which revealed spastic contractions in the distal esophagus and a small hiatal hernia (Fig. 1). She was then referred for high-resolution esophageal manometry (HREM), which demonstrated a normal resting LES pressure and normal integrated relaxation pressure (IRP) but 60% hypercontractile swallows (Fig. 2). As her symptoms were mild to moderate, she was managed conservatively with a PPI and lifestyle modification. However, several years later her symptoms persisted and increased in frequency. She was then started on diltiazem 60 mg four times per day. Initially this improved her symptoms, but they again returned. She was trialed on amitriptyline 25 mg daily and as needed activated charcoal. Over the ensuing years, her symptoms fluctuated, and consistent symptom control was hindered by spotty adherence to her medications.

S. Kamionkowski (✉)
Department of Gastroenterology and Hepatology, Case Western Reserve University School of Medicine, MetroHealth Medical Center, Cleveland, OH, USA
e-mail: skamionkowski@metrohealth.org

© The Author(s), under exclusive license to Springer Nature Switzerland AG 2024
R. Fass et al. (eds.), *Esophageal Disorders*,
https://doi.org/10.1007/978-3-031-56441-3_31

Fig. 1 Fluoroscopic barium swallow showing spastic contractions in the distal esophagus and a small hiatal hernia

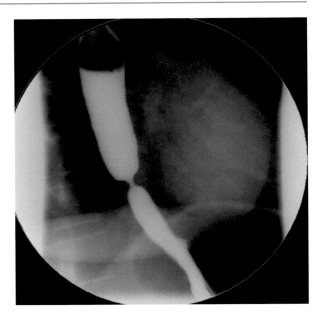

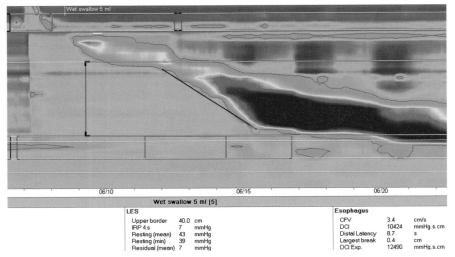

LES				Esophagus		
Upper border	40.0	cm		CFV	3.4	cm/s
IRP 4 s	7	mmHg		DCI	10424	mmHg.s.cm
Resting (mean)	43	mmHg		Distal Latency	8.7	s
Resting (min)	39	mmHg		Largest break	0.4	cm
Residual (mean)	7	mmHg		DCI Exp.	12490	mmHg.s.cm

Fig. 2 Representative swallow from high-resolution esophageal manometry demonstrating a hypercontractile swallow with normal integrated relaxation pressure. The tabular numbers below pertain to this swallow

2   Discussion

Our patient presented with chronic non-cardiac chest pain and was ultimately diagnosed with hypercontractile esophagus, defined as at least 20% of swallows with abnormally high distal contractile integral (DCI >8000 mmHg.s.cm). Esophageal peristalsis was otherwise normal and without evidence of an esophageal outlet obstruction [1]. While some use the term jackhammer esophagus interchangeably with hypercontractile esophagus, jackhammer is in fact one of three recognized subtypes of hypercontractile esophagus differentiated based on the manometric pattern of esophageal contraction [2]. The three subtypes of hypercontractile esophagus recognized by the Chicago Classification version 4.0 working group include the single-peaked, multi-peaked contractions (Jackhammer esophagus), and hypercontractile lower esophageal sphincter [2].

When determining how to manage a patient with hypercontractile esophagus, it is important to consider the symptom character and severity. If the primary symptom is dysphagia, interventions to relax the smooth muscles of the distal esophagus may be more effective, whereas patients such as ours who present with non-cardiac chest pain may find more benefit from neuromodulation. In patients with mild to moderate symptoms, observation and sometimes pharmacologic treatment are recommended, as the disorder can be transient and may not persist on subsequent tests if manometry is repeated [3]. In patients with severe or persistent symptoms, invasive therapies may be more effective, including esophageal botulinum toxin injection, peroral endoscopic myotomy (POEM) with an extended myotomy, and long Heller myotomy. Data supporting these treatments is less robust than with achalasia [4].

References

1. Yadlapati R, Kahrilas PJ, Fox MR, Bredenoord AJ, et al. Esophageal motility disorders on high-resolution manometry: Chicago classification version 4.0©. Neurogastroenterol Motil. 2021 Jan;33(1):e14058. https://doi.org/10.1111/nmo.14058.
2. Chen JW, Savarino E, Smout A, Xiao Y, de Bortoli N, Yadlapati R, Cock C. Chicago classification update (v4.0): technical review on diagnostic criteria for hypercontractile esophagus. Neurogastroenterol Motil. 2021 Jun;33(6):e14115. https://doi.org/10.1111/nmo.14115. Epub 2021 Mar 17
3. Huang L, Pimentel M, Rezaie A. Do Jackhammer contractions lead to achalasia? A longitudinal study. Neurogastroenterol Motil. 2017;29(3). https://doi.org/10.1111/nmo.12953.
4. Valdovinos MA, Zavala-Solares MR, Coss-Adame E. Esophageal hypomotility and spastic motor disorders: current diagnosis and treatment. Curr Gastroenterol Rep. 2014;16(11):421. https://doi.org/10.1007/s11894-014-0421-1.

Reflux After Sleeve Gastrectomy

Josue Davila

1   Case Presentation

A 65-year-old female with a history of fibromyalgia and gastroesophageal reflux disease (GERD) with a history of documented erosive esophagitis and short-segment Barrett's esophagus with indefinite dysplasia, sleeve gastrectomy, anxiety, obstructive sleep apnea and nicotine abuse presented to the clinic for long-standing history of nocturnal reflux symptoms, a hoarse voice, and intermittent dysphagia despite treatment with twice-daily 40 mg esomeprazole. Upper endoscopy showed LA grade B erosive esophagitis (Fig. 1), and 40 mg famotidine at bedtime was added to her therapy. She underwent an upper GI series, which showed a large volume of reflux to the level of the thoracic inlet, as well as a medium-sized sliding-type (type 1) hiatal hernia with sleeve gastrectomy anatomy. A pH impedance test was obtained and showed abnormal esophageal acid exposure in both upright and supine positions despite maximal medical therapy. The patient was referred to a foregut surgeon, and a decision was made to convert her sleeve gastrectomy to Roux-en-Y bypass. The patient had complete resolution of her symptoms after this surgery.

J. Davila (✉)
Division of Hospital Medicine, Cleveland Clinic Foundation, Cleveland, OH, USA
e-mail: davilaj3@ccf.org

© The Author(s), under exclusive license to Springer Nature
Switzerland AG 2024
R. Fass et al. (eds.), *Esophageal Disorders*,
https://doi.org/10.1007/978-3-031-56441-3_32

Fig. 1 Upper endoscopy
showing LA grade B
erosive esophagitis and a
sliding hiatal hernia

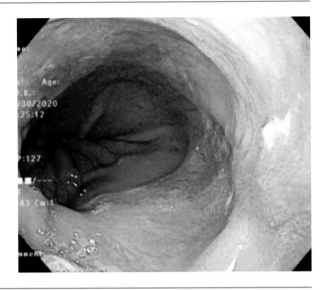

Fig. 1 Upper endoscopy showing LA grade B erosive esophagitis and a sliding hiatal hernia

2 Discussion

With rising prevalence of obesity throughout the world, sleeve gastrectomy is frequently performed [1]. GERD can occur or worsen after sleeve gastrectomy as the smaller and narrower stomach leads to reduced gastric compliance, and this increases the risk of gastroesophageal reflux into the esophagus. The prevalence of GERD after sleeve gastrectomy may range from 5 to 69% [2].

Patients who underwent sleeve gastrectomy are not candidates for traditional antireflux surgery. The best approach to manage refractory GERD with persistent objective evidence of the disease in a patient with prior sleeve gastrectomy is to convert their sleeve gastrectomy to a Roux-en-Y gastric bypass (RYGB), as was done in this patient. RYGB is recognized as a treatment for GERD in obese patients or patients who developed severe, uncontrollable GERD after sleeve gastrectomy [3]. Its efficacy is thought to be multifactorial. RYGB often results in significant weight loss which reduces symptoms of GERD. Furthermore, the small gastric pouch will only produce a small amount of acid compared to the entire stomach prior to surgery. The gastrojejunal bypass also allows for clearance of gastric acid into the small bowel more quickly as it does not need to pass through the pylorus. This also leaves less opportunity for gastroesophageal reflux to occur [3, 4].

References

1. Angrisani L. 2014: the year of the sleeve supremacy. Obes Surg. 2017;27(6):1626–7. https://doi.org/10.1007/s11695-017-2681-y.
2. Coupaye M, Gorbatchef C, Calabrese D, Sami O, Msika S, Coffin B, Ledoux S. Gastroesophageal reflux after sleeve gastrectomy: a prospective mechanistic study. Obes Surg. 2017;28(3):838–45. https://doi.org/10.1007/s11695-017-2942-9.
3. Angrisani L, Santonicola A, Iovino P, et al. Bariatric surgery worldwide 2013. Obes Surg. 2015;25:1822–32. https://doi.org/10.1007/s11695-015-1657-z.
4. Ashrafi D, Osland E, Memon MA. Bariatric surgery and gastroesophageal reflux disease. Ann Transl Med. 2020;8(Suppl 1):S11.

When a Wrap Comes Undone

Josue Davila

1   Case Presentation

A 28-year-old male with a history of spastic paralysis secondary to cerebral palsy and Nissen fundoplication 17 years prior to presentation presented to the clinic for 10 years of persistent postprandial heartburn. The patient denies having dysphagia. An upper endoscopy was performed and showed a slipped Nissen and large hiatal hernia (Fig. 1). The patient's symptoms persisted despite twice-daily proton pump inhibitors (PPI) and H2 receptor antagonist at bedtime. Ultimately, the patient had a high-resolution esophageal manometry (HREM), which showed a normal integrated relaxation pressure (IRP), 20% weak swallows, and 80% failed swallows, as well as a hiatal hernia (Fig. 2). The patient was diagnosed with ineffective esophageal motility and a slipped Nissen fundoplication. Hernia repair with Toupet fundoplication was recommended, but the patient declined.

J. Davila (✉)
Division of Hospital Medicine, Cleveland Clinic Foundation, Cleveland, OH, USA
e-mail: davilaj3@ccf.org

Fig. 1 Upper endoscopy
showing a large hiatal
hernia

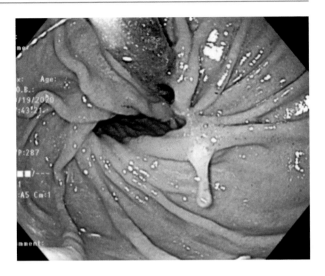

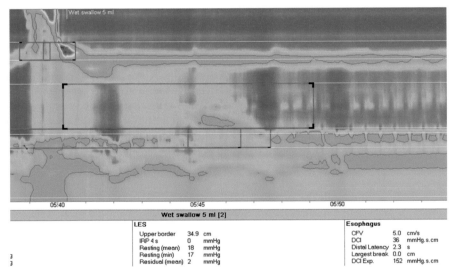

LES			Esophagus		
Upper border	34.9	cm	CFV	5.0	cm/s
IRP 4 s	0	mmHg	DCI	36	mmHg.s.cm
Resting (mean)	18	mmHg	Distal Latency	2.3	s
Resting (min)	17	mmHg	Largest break	0.0	cm
Residual (mean)	2	mmHg	DCI Exp.	152	mmHg.s.cm

Fig. 2 Representative swallow from high-resolution esophageal manometry showing a failed swallow with normal integrated relaxation pressure. Tabular numbers below represent this particular swallow

2 Discussion

Most patients with GERD can be effectively treated with lifestyle modifications and PPIs. However, a subset of patients developed persistent symptoms despite maximal treatment and may require antireflux surgery. While Nissen fundoplication is a highly successful antireflux surgery, the fundoplication can become displaced in up to 7–20% of the time [1–3]. Another potential side effect of surgical fundoplication is postoperative persistent dysphagia, which occurs in 3–24% of patients [4, 5]. The risk of postoperative dysphagia is increased in patients who have impaired esophageal peristalsis prior to surgery. For this reason, HREM is often performed prior to antireflux surgery, and partial rather than complete fundoplication is recommended in patients with impaired esophageal peristalsis. A maneuver called "multiple rapid swallows," in which the patient takes several small sips in quick succession during the HREM, can help determine whether the patient has enough peristaltic reserve to tolerate a fundoplication without developing dysphagia. Patients with an adequate peristaltic reserve as demonstrated by an increase in contractile vigor after the multiple rapid swallows remain candidates for surgical fundoplication.

References

1. Hashemi M, Peters JH, DeMeester TR, et al. Laparoscopic repair of large type III hiatal hernia: objective followup reveals high recurrence rate. J Am Coll Surg. 2000;190:553–60.
2. Floch NR, Hinder RA, Klingler PJ, et al. Is laparoscopic reoperation for failed antireflux surgery feasible? Arch Surg. 1999;134(7):733–7.
3. Mattar SG, Bowers SP, Galloway KD, et al. Long-term outcome of laparoscopic repair of paraesophageal hernia. Surg Endosc. 2002;16:745–9.
4. Alexander HC, Hendler RS, Seymour NE, Shires GT. Laparoscopic treatment of gastroesophageal reflux disease. Am Surg. 1997;63:434–44.
5. Anvari M, Allen CJ. Prospective evaluation of dysphagia before and after laparoscopic Nissen fundoplication without routine division of short gastrics. Surg Laparosc Endosc. 1996;6:424–9.

Paraesophageal Hernia Causing a Blockage

Josue Davila

1 Case Presentation

A 27-year-old female with a history of morbid obesity, thyroidectomy, and smoking presented to clinic for regurgitation of solids associated with chest pain for 1 year. The pain is sharp, located at the lower end of the sternum, and most prominent after eating or drinking. Her symptoms have progressed and increased in frequency and now occur after any ingestion of solids or liquids. She has lost 20 pounds since the onset of symptoms. The patient denies odynophagia, hematemesis, or abdominal pain. Omeprazole 20 mg daily and sucralfate three times per day did not improve her symptoms. A chest X-ray showed moderate- to large-size hiatal hernia. An upper endoscopy was performed and demonstrated a moderate-size paraesophageal hernia (Fig. 1). There was no esophagitis or any other esophageal abnormalities. A pH impedance test was also performed with no pathologic acid exposure and negative symptom indices. High-resolution esophageal manometry (HREM) showed normal peristalsis with an elevated integrated relaxation pressure (IRP) (Fig. 2). The IRP remained elevated in the supine and upright positions, consistent with esophagogastric junction outlet obstruction (EGJOO). It is likely that the patient's EGJOO was due to paraesophageal hernia. She was eventually referred for surgical evaluation for hernia repair and underwent a laparoscopic repair of her paraesophageal hernia with significant postoperative improvement in her dysphagia and postprandial pain.

J. Davila (✉)

Division of Hospital Medicine, Cleveland Clinic Foundation, Cleveland, OH, USA

e-mail: davilaj3@ccf.org

R. Fass et al. (eds.), *Esophageal Disorders*,

https://doi.org/10.1007/978-3-031-56441-3_34

Fig. 1 Upper endoscopy demonstrating a moderate sized paraesophageal hernia

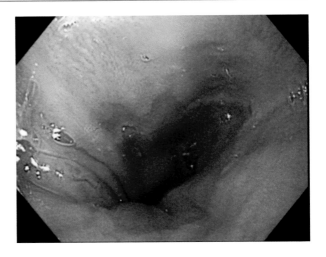

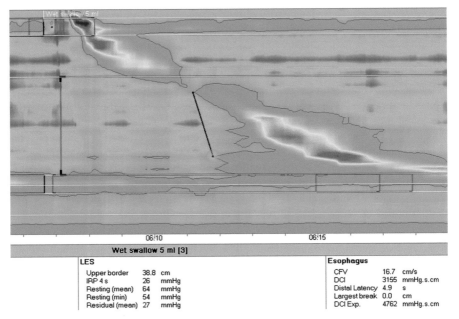

LES			Esophagus		
Upper border	38.8	cm	CFV	16.7	cm/s
IRP 4 s	26	mmHg	DCI	3155	mmHg.s.cm
Resting (mean)	64	mmHg	Distal Latency	4.9	s
Resting (min)	54	mmHg	Largest break	0.0	cm
Residual (mean)	27	mmHg	DCI Exp.	4762	mmHg.s.cm

Fig. 2 Representative swallow from high-resolution esophageal manometry demonstrating normal peristalsis with an elevated integrated relaxation pressure. Tabular numbers below pertain to this swallow

2   Discussion

The most common presenting symptoms of EGJOO are dysphagia (seen in up to 75% of patients) and regurgitation (up to 73% of cases), which were experienced by the patient [1]. Chest pain and heartburn are other common symptoms [1, 2]. This patient case is consistent with the Chicago Classification 4.0 (CCv4.0) criteria for EGJOO which include an elevated IRP in both supine and upright positions [3]. When EGJOO is diagnosed, secondary causes should be ruled out, such as hiatal hernia, esophageal web or stricture, esophageal candidiasis, neoplasms, and possible infiltrative diseases [2, 3]. In our case, the cause of the EGJOO is suspected to be secondary to the paraesophageal hernia. Our patient presented with severe symptoms including frequent dysphagia and significant weight loss. These justify an aggressive approach to management, which is why our patient was referred for corrective surgery. In the absence of a secondary cause, patients with severe or persistent symptoms should have confirmation of clinically significant obstruction by a timed barium esophagram or EndoFLIP. When appropriate, patients with EGJOO and no anatomical abnormality can then be treated with pneumatic dilation, peroral endoscopic myotomy (POEM), or botulinum toxin injection at the lower esophageal sphincter [2, 3].

References

1. Beveridge C, Lynch K. Diagnosis and management of esophagogastric junction outflow obstruction. Gastroenterol Hepatol (N Y). 2020;16(3):131–8.
2. Samo S, Qayed E. Esophagogastric junction outflow obstruction: where are we now in diagnosis and management? World J Gastroenterol. 2019;25(4):411–7.
3. Yadlapati R, Kahrilas PJ, Fox MR, Bredenoord AJ, et al. Esophageal motility disorders on high-resolution manometry: Chicago classification version 4.0©. Neurogastroenterol Motil. 2021;33(1):e14058.

Chronic Cough and Spastic Contractions

Josue Davila

1   Case Presentation

A 75-year-old female with a history of obesity, hypertension, and obstructive sleep apnea presented to the gastroenterology clinic for 10 years of chronic productive cough and epigastric abdominal pain not responsive to intermittent use of esomeprazole. Her symptoms were worst at night and were associated with eating. However, the patient was unable to identify a specific type of food that exacerbates the symptoms. She had not lost weight or had a decrease in her appetite. She followed a specific diet with no chocolate, caffeine, or tomato-based products. An upper endoscopy was obtained and showed a 4 cm hiatal hernia with a dilated and tortuous distal esophagus (Fig. 1). Subsequently the patient underwent high-resolution esophageal manometry (HREM), which showed 30% weak swallows, 20% normal swallows, 50% swallows with a short distal latency, and normal integrated relaxation pressure (IRP), consistent with distal esophageal spasm (Fig. 2). A timed barium esophagram was performed, which showed mildly distended tortuous distal esophagus and complete esophageal emptying of the barium column by 2 min. She was diagnosed with distal esophageal spasm and was offered Botox injection into the distal esophagus. However, the patient declined invasive therapy and decided to focus on dietary modifications: small sips and bites to limit symptoms. She was also started on esomeprazole 40 mg twice daily. She reported mild improvement of symptoms.

J. Davila (✉)
Division of Hospital Medicine, Cleveland Clinic Foundation, Cleveland, OH, USA
e-mail: davilaj3@ccf.org

© The Author(s), under exclusive license to Springer Nature Switzerland AG 2024
R. Fass et al. (eds.), *Esophageal Disorders*,
https://doi.org/10.1007/978-3-031-56441-3_35

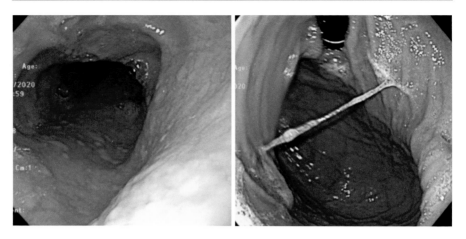

Fig. 1 Upper endoscopy showing a 4 cm hiatal hernia with a dilated and tortuous distal esophagus

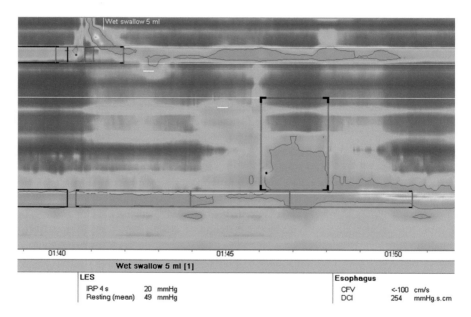

Fig. 2 Representative swallow from high-resolution esophageal manometry demonstrating a high integrated relaxation pressure and a simultaneous spastic contraction of the distal esophagus. Tabular numbers below pertain to this swallow

2   Discussion

Distal esophageal spasm (DES) is an uncommon esophageal motility disorder characterized by premature contractions of the distal esophagus. Monometrically this is confirmed with at least 20% of swallows having a short distal latency [1]. DES may present with dysphagia, chest pain, or GERD symptoms [2]. The diagnosis is confirmed by HREM. EndoFLIP can support the diagnosis, as it may show repetitive retrograde contractions [1, 2].

Treatment of DES begins with ruling out secondary causes such as uncontrolled GERD, opiate use, and obstruction at the esophageal outlet. Patients' management depends on symptom severity. Patients with mild to moderate symptoms should be managed conservatively as the disorder can be transient at times. It is often appropriate to repeat HREM 6 months following the initial diagnosis to confirm the persistence of the disorder.

Furthermore, it is important to differentiate transit symptoms such as dysphagia from perceptive symptoms such as chest pain. Dysphagia may be best treated with smooth muscle relaxants, while chest pain may be best treated with neuromodulators, though evidence to support this distinction is lacking. Our patient's epigastric pain may have been a perceptive symptom of DES, while her chronic cough could have been an obstructive symptom of DES or related to GERD. GERD may also represent a secondary cause of DES in this patient, and thus initial management can focus on treatment of GERD, as was done in this patient. Further treatment was declined by our patient, but adding a tricyclic antidepressant would have been a reasonable noninvasive next step given her complaint of a perceptive symptom. Reflux testing off PPI treatment to evaluate for GERD or other esophageal disorders could also be pursued in this patient.

References

1. Almansa C, Heckman MG, Devault KR, Bouras E, Achem SR. Esophageal spasm: demographic, clinical, radiographic, and manometric features in 108 patients. Dis Esophagus. 2011;25(3):214–21.
2. Khalaf M, Chowdhary S, Elias PS, Castell D. Distal esophageal spasm: a review. Am J Med. 2018;131(9):1034–40.

Is It Achalasia?

Erika Mengalle

1   Case Presentation

A 57-year-old male with gigantism, hypertension, and atrial fibrillation presented to the gastroenterology clinic for difficulty swallowing for 1 year. He described a choking sensation when swallowing both solids and liquids, with the urge to regurgitate the food but without coughing or becoming short of breath. His symptoms had progressively worsened to the point where he was experiencing this with every meal. He had lost his appetite and lost 30 lbs. over the course of the year. He denied heartburn, nausea, vomiting, or abdominal pain. A barium swallow study done just prior to presentation showed a dilated esophagus with a bird's beak appearance of the distal esophagus and severely diminished intrathoracic esophageal peristalsis (Fig. 1). Esophagogastroduodenoscopy (EGD) was performed, which revealed normal-appearing esophageal mucosa, unremarkable esophageal biopsies, and no resistance at the esophagogastric junction (EGJ) (Fig. 2). He then underwent high-resolution esophageal manometry (HREM), which showed a normal integrated relaxation pressure (IRP) of 13 mmHg, with 100% failed swallows, 50% with pan-pressurization of the esophagus (Fig. 3). These findings were suspicious for type 2 achalasia, but further confirmation was required given the normal IRP. A timed barium esophagram showed slight narrowing of the esophagus at the GEJ. Mild esophageal residual was noted at 0 and 1 min that was emptied within 2 min (Fig. 4). He also reported an additional 40 lbs. weight loss. He then underwent an EGD with endoluminal functional lumen imaging probe (EndoFLIP), which revealed a low distensibility index and no antegrade or retrograde repetitive esophageal contractions (Fig. 5). A presumptive diagnosis of type 2 achalasia was made. Given the

E. Mengalle (✉)
Lifespan Physician Group, Division of Hospital Medicine, Warren Alpert Medical School of Brown University, Rhode Island Hospital, Providence, RI, USA
e-mail: emengalle@lifespan.org

© The Author(s), under exclusive license to Springer Nature
Switzerland AG 2024
R. Fass et al. (eds.), *Esophageal Disorders*,
https://doi.org/10.1007/978-3-031-56441-3_36

Fig. 1 Barium swallow
showing a dilated
esophagus with a bird's
beak appearance

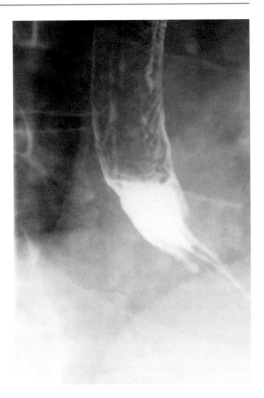

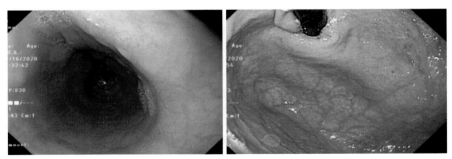

Fig. 2 Endoscopy showing a normal esophagus and gastroesophageal junction

severity of his symptoms with significant weight loss, he was referred for a peroral
endoscopic myotomy (POEM). His symptoms markedly improved postoperatively.

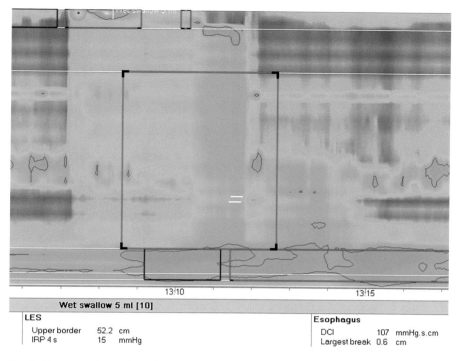

LES			Esophagus		
Upper border	52.2	cm	DCI	107	mmHg.s.cm
IRP 4 s	15	mmHg	Largest break	0.6	cm

Fig. 3 Representative swallow from high-resolution esophageal manometry demonstrating a normal integrated relaxation pressure with pan-pressurization of the esophagus

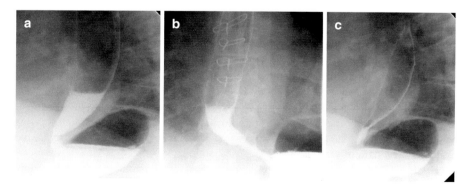

Fig. 4 Timed barium esophagram showing narrowing of the esophagus at the GEJ. Also, mild esophageal residual contrast was noted at 0 (**a**) and 1 (**b**) minute that was emptied within 2 min (**c**)

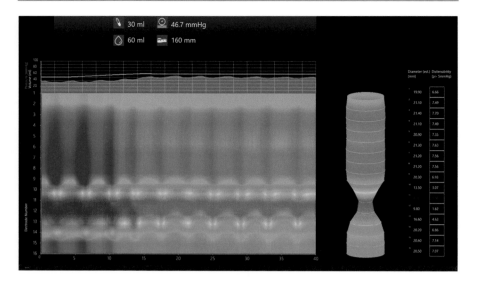

Fig. 5 Endoluminal functional lumen imaging probe results showing a low distensibility index and no antegrade or retrograde repetitive esophageal contractions

2   Discussion

It is sometimes difficult to distinguish absent contractility from achalasia. Both disorders may initially present with symptoms of dysphagia, heartburn, and weight loss. The primary modality used for diagnosis is HREM. While in both disorders, there is a complete failure of peristalsis, the defining factor is the elevated IRP (>15 mmHg) seen in achalasia versus a normal IRP in absent contractility. However, a borderline IRP (10–15 mmHg) can be seen in some subtypes of achalasia [1, 2]. As such, patients with equivocal findings on HREM require further evaluation to elicit abnormal function typically with timed barium esophagram and/or endoluminal functional lumen imaging probe (EndoFLIP). In this case, the timed barium esophagram was non-revealing, but the EndoFLIP results supported the diagnosis of achalasia. Given the patient's symptom severity and the evidence supporting achalasia, a decision was made to proceed with POEM which subsequently improved the patient's symptoms.

EndoFLIP is used as a complementary tool when manometrsy and barium esophagram findings are equivocal or normal in symptomatic patients. While manometry measures the static pressure through the esophagogastric junction (EGJ), EndoFLIP is able to measure the radial force through resistance to distension, which is termed distensibility [3, 4]. This provides a different modality for measurement of real-time EGJ distensibility, which often provides important an added data point when attempting to diagnose disorders of the esophageal outlet. EndoFLIP has also been used to predict response to interventions that affect the EGJ comparing pre- and post-intervention measurements.

References

1. Kahrilas PJ, Bredenoord AJ, et al. The Chicago classification of esophageal motility disorders, v3.0. Neurogastroenterol Motil. 2015;27:160–74. https://doi.org/10.1111/nmo.12477.
2. Carlson DA, Pandolfino JE. High-resolution manometry in clinical practice. Gastroenterol Hepatol (N Y). 2015;11(6):374–84.
3. Ata-Lawenko RM, Lee YY. Emerging roles of the endolumenal functional lumen imaging probe in gastrointestinal motility disorders. J Neurogastroenterol Motil. 2017;23(2):164–70. https://doi.org/10.5056/jnm16171.
4. Donnan EN, Pandolfino JE. EndoFLIP in the esophagus: assessing sphincter function, wall stiffness, and motility to guide treatment. Gastroenterol Clin N Am. 2020;49(3):427–35. https://doi.org/10.1016/j.gtc.2020.04.002.

Is It Achalasia or Absent Contractility?

Erika Mengalle

1 Case Presentation

A 43-year-old female with hypertension and hyperlipidemia presented to the gastroenterology clinic for 1 year of dysphagia to liquids and solids. The food was getting stuck at the level of the sternum. Occasionally she would regurgitate undigested food. Symptoms were progressing and at the time of presentation, were occurring daily. She was unable to tolerate any medications and had decreased her food intake though she had not lost weight. She also reported epigastric pain exacerbated by eating and accompanied by nausea and vomiting. The patient had initially been seen by her primary care provider who referred her for an endoscopy. The esophageal anatomy was normal with biopsies negative for eosinophilic esophagitis (Fig. 1). She then underwent high-resolution esophageal manometry (HREM) which showed 100% failed swallows and a median Integrated relaxation pressure (IRP) near the upper limit of normal (Fig. 2). There was suspicion for achalasia but the diagnosis was not confirmed. The patient was referred for a timed barium esophagram, which showed 40% retention of contrast after 5 min, increasing suspicion for achalasia (Fig. 3). In order to clarify the diagnosis, the patient was referred for repeat EGD with endoscopic functional lumen imaging probe (EndoFLIP), which showed a dilated non-peristaltic esophagus with a tight esophagogastric junction (EGJ) (Fig. 4) and a low distensibility index with absent contractions (Fig. 5). Given these confirmatory findings of achalasia, she was referred to surgery for peroral endoscopic myotomy procedure (POEM) with improvement in her symptoms (Table 1).

E. Mengalle (✉)
Lifespan Physician Group, Division of Hospital Medicine, Warren Alpert Medical School of Brown University, Rhode Island Hospital, Providence, RI, USA
e-mail: emengalle@lifespan.org

© The Author(s), under exclusive license to Springer Nature Switzerland AG 2024
R. Fass et al. (eds.), *Esophageal Disorders*,
https://doi.org/10.1007/978-3-031-56441-3_37

149

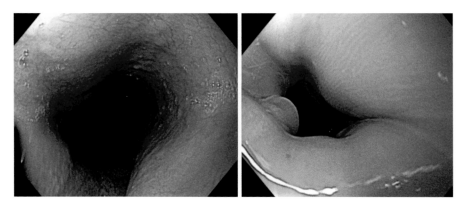

Fig. 1 Normal upper endoscopy

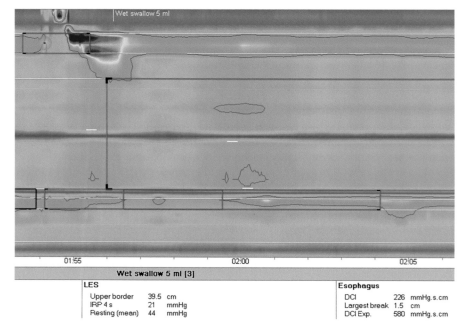

LES			Esophagus		
Upper border	39.5	cm	DCI	226	mmHg.s.cm
IRP 4 s	21	mmHg	Largest break	1.5	cm
Resting (mean)	44	mmHg	DCI Exp.	580	mmHg.s.cm

Fig. 2 Representative swallow from high-resolution esophageal manometry showing a failed swallow with borderline integrated relaxation pressure. Tabular numbers below represent this particular swallow

Fig. 3 Timed barium esophagram showing retention of contrast after 5 min

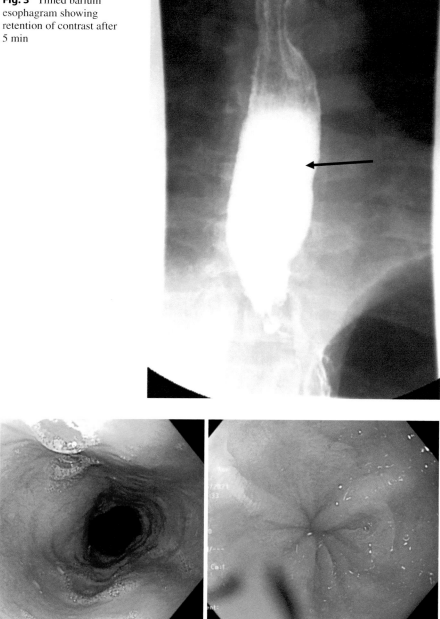

Fig. 4 Upper endoscopy showing a dilated esophagus with tight EGJ

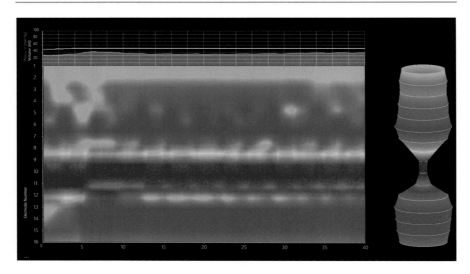

Fig. 5 Endoscopic functional lumen imaging probe images showing no contractile activity and a tight LES with low distensibility

Table 1 EndoFlip results pre-POEM and Post-POEM, showing a large increase in distensibility index indicating a successful myotomy

Balloon pressure (mmHg)	Diameter (mm)	Distensibility index
Pre-POEM		
40	4.7	1.1
50	4.9	1.0
60	6.0	1.0
Post-POEM		
40	10.7	5.8
50	12.4	6.0
60	14.3	5.5

2 Discussion

Achalasia is an esophageal motility disorder characterized by a non-relaxing lower esophageal sphincter (LES) and lack of organized peristalsis. It is an uncommon cause of dysphagia, with an incidence of 1.6 cases in 100,000 individuals [1]. It results from a degeneration of inhibitory ganglion cells in the esophageal myenteric plexus leading to impaired relaxation of the LES [2].

After ruling out pseudoachalasia with an esophagogastroduodenoscopy (EGD), the gold standard for diagnosing achalasia is HREM. Occasionally, the diagnosis of achalasia is not clear after HREM, especially if the IRP is normal, or just slightly elevated. In these cases, adjunctive tests are recommended to confirm the diagnosis. These include a timed barium esophagram, which can be used to show esophageal retention of barium at timed intervals. EndoFLIP is another supportive test, which measures distensibility and cross-sectional area across the LES [2, 3]. In our case all of these tests were used to confirm the diagnosis of achalasia with a degree of confidence that was high enough to refer the patient for an invasive but effective treatment.

While there is no cure for achalasia, the three definitive therapies are pneumatic dilatation, Heller myotomy with partial fundoplication, and peroral esophageal myotomy (POEM). Our patient elected the latter and did well post-procedure.

References

1. Sadowski DC, Ackah F, Jiang B, Svenson LW. Achalasia: incidence, prevalence and survival. A population-based study. Neurogastroenterol Motil. 2010;22(9):e256.
2. Ates F, Vaezi MF. The pathogenesis and management of achalasia: current status and future directions. Gut Liver. 2015;9(4):449–63.
3. Vaezi F, Pandolfino JE, et al. ACG clinical guidelines: diagnosis and management of achalasia. AJG. 2020;115(9):1393–411.

But, Is There an Actual Blockage?

Erika Mengalle

1   Case Presentation

A 64-year-old female with coronary artery disease and type 2 diabetes mellitus presented to the gastroenterology clinic for 10 years of persistent daily dysphagia to solids and pills. An esophagogastroduodenoscopy (EGD) was obtained and showed a normal esophagus without a stricture or mass. A barium esophagram was then performed and showed thickening at the gastric cardia. EGD was repeated, but this was again unremarkable, and biopsies were negative for eosinophilic esophagitis. Her symptoms persisted despite compliance with high-dose proton pump inhibitor (PPI) therapy.

The patient was then referred for high-resolution esophageal manometry (HREM), which showed high integrated relaxation pressure (IRP) of 29 mmHg with 40% failed swallows and 20% weak swallows in the supine position. Additional five swallows in the upright position also showed elevated IRP, all consistent with esophagogastric junction outlet obstruction (EGJOO) (Fig. 1). Endoscopic ultrasound (EUS) was performed, which showed an unremarkable esophagogastric junction (EGJ). She was managed conservatively, but her symptoms persisted over the ensuing year. HREM was then repeated, and this time showed an elevated IRP with 10% weak swallows and 60% of the swallows with premature contractions (Fig. 2). She was referred for a timed barium esophagogram, which revealed a bird beak appearance and dilated distal esophagus without clearance of pooled contrast within 5 min (Fig. 3). As the nature of her motility disorder remained incompletely defined, she underwent upper endoscopy with endoscopic functional lumen imaging probe (EndoFLIP), which demonstrated a low EGJ diameter, low distensibility index, and

E. Mengalle (✉)
Lifespan Physician Group, Division of Hospital Medicine, Warren Alpert Medical School of
Brown University, Rhode Island Hospital, Providence, RI, USA
e-mail: emengalle@lifespan.org

© The Author(s), under exclusive license to Springer Nature
Switzerland AG 2024
R. Fass et al. (eds.), *Esophageal Disorders*,
https://doi.org/10.1007/978-3-031-56441-3_38

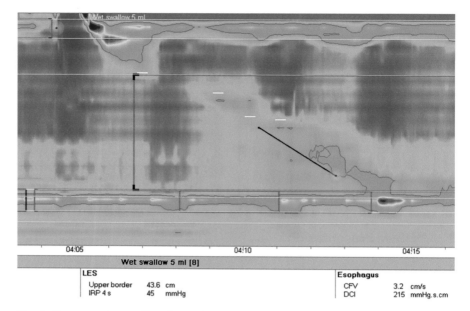

Fig. 1 Representative swallow from high-resolution esophageal manometry showing a weak swallow with a high integrated relaxation pressure. Tabular numbers below are representative of this particular swallow

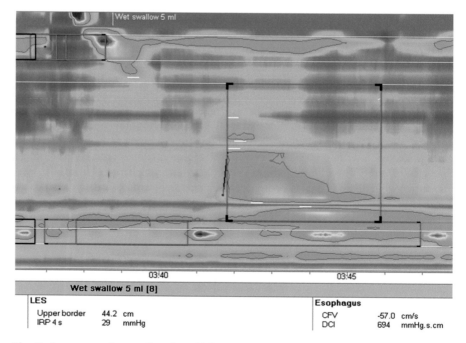

Fig. 2 A representative swallow from high-resolution esophageal manometry demonstrating a weak swallow with a simultaneous contraction of the distal esophagus and an elevated integrated relaxation pressure. Tabular numbers below are representative of this particular swallow

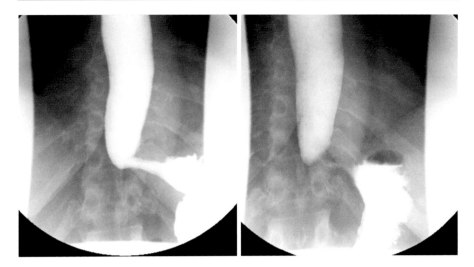

Fig. 3 Timed barium esophagram revealing a bird beak appearance (left image) and lack of clearance of pooled contrast within 5 min (right image)

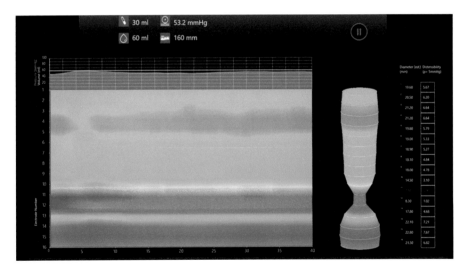

Fig. 4 EndoFLIP showing a low EGJ diameter, low distensibility index (DI), and absence of esophageal contractions, consistent with achalasia. No repetitive antegrade or retrograde contractions were noted

absence of any type of esophageal contractions (Fig. 4). Balloon dilation of the gastroesophageal junction was performed, but the patient had no relief of her symptoms. Given the persistence of her symptoms and EndoFLIP findings, the patient ultimately underwent peroral endoscopic myotomy (POEM) and experienced resolution of her symptoms after the procedure.

2   Discussion

Our patient presented with persistent symptoms of dysphagia with a dysfunction of the esophageal outlet. However, her final diagnosis remains unclear. Her initial HREM suggested EGJOO alone, while the second HREM showed EGJOO with overlapping distal esophageal spasm. A subsequent EndoFLIP showed findings typical of achalasia. At times, the differentiation between achalasia and EGJOO with an additional overlapping esophageal motility disorder can be subtle. In this setting, supportive tests such as timed barium esophagram and/or EndoFLIP can be used as adjunctive measures to clarify the diagnosis. EndoFLIP is a novel tool that measures the intraluminal diameter and pressures during volumetric distension of the sphincter, which gives a real-time assessment of the esophagogastric function [1]. It can also assess secondary peristalsis in real time, and the contraction pattern can support or negate the diagnosis of achalasia [2].

While the initial management of EGJOO is typically conservative, especially in the absence of severe symptoms, invasive interventions at the LES can be considered when the symptoms and diagnosis are persistent. In these cases, treatment of EGJOO and achalasia can be similar and involve POEM, pneumatic dilation, or surgical myotomy. In our case, POEM would be a reasonable treatment choice whether the diagnosis is achalasia or EGJOO. In this case, the patient had a positive response to the therapeutic intervention.

References

1. Cha B, Jung KW. Diagnosis of dysphagia: high resolution manometry & endoFLIP. Korean J Gastroenterol. 2021;77(2):64–70. Korean. https://doi.org/10.4166/kjg.2021.018.
2. Carlson DA, Lin Z, Kahrilas PJ, et al. The functional lumen imaging probe detects esophageal contractility not observed with manometry in patients with achalasia. Gastroenterology. 2015;149(7):1742–51. https://doi.org/10.1053/j.gastro.2015.08.005.

Stuck in the Middle

Erika Mengalle

1 Case Presentation

A 34-year-old male with hypertension and tobacco use presented to the gastroenterology clinic for 4 years of dysphagia that had progressively worsened over the last 2 years. He described difficulty swallowing initially with solids which then progressed to both liquids and solids, as well as regurgitation that interfered with his sleep. He denied abdominal pain, nausea, vomiting, and weight loss. He underwent an esophagogastroduodenoscopy (EGD), which showed a dilated esophagus with resistance in traversing the lower esophageal sphincter (LES) (Fig. 1). Esophageal biopsies were negative for eosinophilic esophagitis. Unfortunately, the patient could not tolerate the placement of a manometry catheter, so high-resolution esophageal manometry was not performed. A timed barium esophagram was obtained demonstrating a dilated aperistaltic esophagus with bird beak appearance and retained contrast in the distal esophagus, 20% of which emptied between 0 and 5 min (Fig. 2). He was then referred for an upper endoscopy with functional lumen imaging probe (FLIP). EndoFLIP revealed a low EGJ diameter, low distensibility index, and absence of esophageal contractions, consistent with achalasia (Fig. 3). He ultimately underwent a peroral endoscopic myotomy (POEM) procedure with improvement in his symptoms.

E. Mengalle (✉)
Lifespan Physician Group, Division of Hospital Medicine, Warren Alpert Medical School of Brown University, Rhode Island Hospital, Providence, RI, USA
e-mail: emengalle@lifespan.org

© The Author(s), under exclusive license to Springer Nature Switzerland AG 2024
R. Fass et al. (eds.), *Esophageal Disorders*,
https://doi.org/10.1007/978-3-031-56441-3_39

159

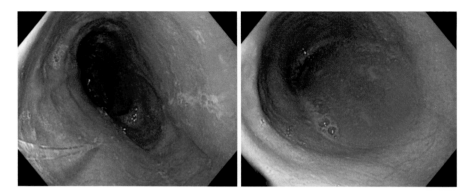

Fig. 1 Upper endoscopy showing a dilated esophagus

Fig. 2 Timed barium
esophagram with bird beak
appearance consistent with
achalasia

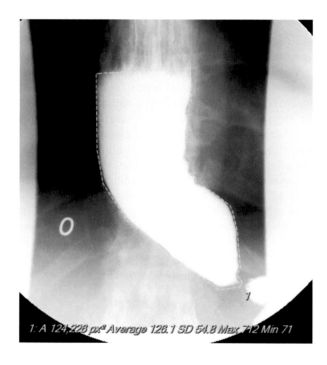

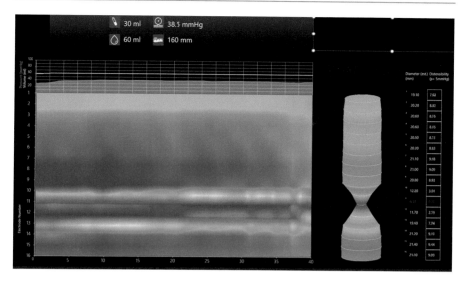

Fig. 3 EndoFLIP showing a low EGJ diameter, low distensibility index (DI), and absence of esophageal contractions, consistent with achalasia

2 Discussion

The gold standard for the diagnosis of achalasia is high-resolution esophageal manometry (HREM) [1]. However, the HREM procedure can be difficult for some patients to tolerate. In situations such as our case, it is sometimes necessary to rely on other testing modalities to make the diagnosis of achalasia. These can include EGD, timed barium esophagram, and EndoFLIP. EndoFLIP is a relatively new technology that measures luminal diameter and pressures during controlled volumetric distension [2]. This recorded pressure, known as distensibility, provides a real-time measurement of EGJ contraction and relaxation. In our case, the EGD revealed findings consistent with achalasia, such as tightness at the LES, a dilated distal esophagus, and retained food contents in the stomach. The timed barium swallow also showed the classic bird beak appearance and confirmed a significant delay in bolus clearance to the stomach. EndoFLIP confirmed a non-relaxing LES and a lack of peristaltic contractions in the esophagus. Between the three tests, a clinician can be confident in the diagnosis of achalasia even without the HREM.

References

1. Chuah SK, Lim CS, Liang CM, et al. Bridging the gap between advancements in the evolution of diagnosis and treatment towards better outcomes in achalasia. Biomed Res Int. 2019;2019:8549187. Published 2019 Feb 6. https://doi.org/10.1155/2019/8549187.
2. Carlson DA, Lin Z, Kahrilas PJ, et al. The functional lumen imaging probe detects esophageal contractility not observed with manometry in patients with achalasia. Gastroenterology. 2015;149(7):1742–51. https://doi.org/10.1053/j.gastro.2015.08.005.

Index